The Mamma Mia! Diet

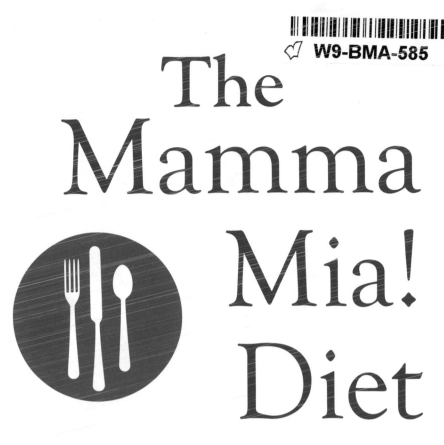

THE SECRET ITALIAN WAY TO GOOD HEALTH

Dr. Paola Lovisetti Scamihorn
& Paola Palestini, PhD

Hatherleigh Press is committed to preserving and protecting the natural resources of the earth. Environmentally responsible and sustainable practices are embraced within the company's mission statement.

Visit us at www.hatherleighpress.com and register online for free offers, discounts, special events, and more.

The Mamma Mia! Diet

Text copyright © 2018 Paola Lovisetti Scamihorn and Paola Palestini

Library of Congress Cataloging-in-Publication Data

is available upon request.

ISBN: 978-1-578-267-323

Cover and Interior Design by Carolyn Kasper

Printed in the United States

10 9 8 7 6 5 4 3 2 1

CONTENTS

Part I:
The Principles of the Mamma Mia! Diet

Part II:
Top Tips for Success

Part III:
Recipes and Seasonal Menus

PREFACE

WO PAOLAS. BUT IT'S not just our names that we have in common; we also share a background, training, and true passion and love for a healthy lifestyle based on simple, frugal food such as fruits, vegetables, legumes, pelagic fish, small amount of meat (especially poultry or rabbit), eggs, and olive oil, all accompanied with semi-sweet desserts. In a few words—the Mamma Mia Diet (MMD). Now, we'd like to take this opportunity to say a few words on why we wrote this book.

The expression "Mamma mia!" immediately brings to mind Italy—the country where you eat good food, drink tasty wine, and stay healthy and in shape. In other words, the Italian lifestyle!

This is not a diet book in the traditional sense. It should instead be considered a useful manual about the Mediterranean diet, a how-to for the Italian style of healthy eating and living, which provides you with all sorts of physical and mental benefits. This is a book you can easily take along with you wherever you go, or use in your own kitchen to prepare nutritious and tasty dishes for yourself and your family.

When Paola Palestini and I created this book, we relied not only on years of personal experience in the field of nutrition, chemistry, and healthy cooking, but also our passion to encourage people to learn how to enjoy the best of Italian life, make positive lifestyle choices, feel better, and live longer. It is our hope that, by learning to establish a positive relationship with wholesome food, you'll be happier—and even **lose some extra pounds** or **maintain normal**

weight. Let good food be your "medicine;" learn to recognize and love it, and it will love you back!

Good food has always been part of my life. I grew up in a very traditional Italian family where fresh, seasonal, and homemade foods were always part of our diet. Cooking has always been one of my passions, even if I chose to become a pharmacist and medical researcher. (Though, since cooking and nutrition are both based on chemistry, my professional expertise has actually helped me better understand how to cook and eat healthily!)

When I was a little girl, I spent a lot of time in the kitchen cooking with my mother (making a big mess!) and learning delicious, traditional recipes using authentic, fresh ingredients and preparing everything from scratch. I still remember preparing *lasagne* or *ravioli* for Christmas, making *crostata* with seasonal fruits for our Sunday lunch, and savoring the smell of homemade fresh bread; the scent was like perfume. This is the way we Italians learn to cook, generation to generation, through daily practice. And in the Italian tradition, I continue this with my kids today.

My dearest wish is that this book should invite you, my readers, not just to experience the *taste* of Italian cooking in a restaurant somewhere in Italy or abroad in your own country, but to *cook*, and to take on an active role by re-proposing the essence of *doing*, the capability of cooking to "create a home" and the need to return to the times and methods of a more relaxed way of life. To dedicate one's efforts to the care of oneself, family, and others—the healthy Italian lifestyle.

—Paola Lovisetti Scamihorn

Having been born in Genoa, Cristoforo Colombo's seaside hometown, I have always been interested in understanding how things worked—especially how *life* works. I grew fond of biology and in particular, the molecular mechanism that makes life possible.

And what is the most complex living organism on earth today? Surely, the human being. This is the reason why I have felt drawn to study biochemistry, the science which studies the chemistry of life, a bridge between biology and chemistry to explain the complex chemical reactions that give birth to life. It is the purview of biochemistry to analyze the structure and transformations of cell components such as proteins, carbohydrates, lipids, nucleic acids, and biomolecules, all while trying to determine how different macronutrients are processed by the body to yield energy.

I am currently a biochemistry professor, and for many years I have been teaching my medical students that each pathology is caused by a biochemical modification of cellular signaling, and that through nutrition, we can introduce a relevant number of molecules and/or macronutrients that can activate positive or negative mechanisms by interacting with our body.

Nutrition is a condition of balance. All the nutrients (both macro and micro) in our food must be introduced in the right amount so that they can act synergistically and have a healthy effect on our body/health. We must not demonize certain nutrients, like carbohydrates or sugars; all of them, in the right amounts, play an important role in our body.

Throughout the history of humanity, it is the right combinations of foods that have made the evolution of humans (and, consequently, of civilization) possible.

What I have tried to do in this book, both by relying on my biochemical knowledge and by compiling other researchers' scientific data and large scale epidemiological investigations, is to explain why a certain molecule has a positive effect, whereas another one, which only differs in small chemical characteristics, can have negative effects.

My hope is that by doing so, I can help bring readers into closer alignment with the ideal balance of nutrients that has helped humanity grow and flourish throughout the centuries.

—Paola Palestini

INTRODUCTION:

Why the Mamma Mia! Diet is Superior to Other Diets

NOWADAYS, WE ARE EXPOSED to any number of diets, each invented by a so-called nutrition guru, each promising easy weight loss in no time at all. Just a few simple changes, they claim, will get us into perfect shape, toned and in good health. The one thing these diets have in common (besides unsustainable results) is that they are monotonous, unrewarding, and even unhealthy, due to being incomplete or difficult to follow. That's why it's always smarter and better in the long run to adopt a healthy lifestyle rather than some crash-course diet. Simple, sustainable changes to one's diet—changes that are relatively easy to follow, beneficial, and can be easily implemented into your way of life—are the key to improved health and well-being.

But what changes should you be making?

Studies have consistently shown that Italians are some of the longest-living people in the world. Just this year, in the northern area of Piedmont, the oldest living person in the world and the last survivor of the 19*th* century passed away at the age of 117. And she is no fluke; her sisters lived to be 100 and 102 themselves! In southern Italy, there are several villages that are called "villages of eternal youth" because of the high numbers of active 100+ year-olds.

The secret to this reproducible longevity lies in their healthy lifestyle: the Mediterranean diet. The Mediterranean Diet, classified by Ancel Keys and part of UNESCO's Intangible Cultural Heritage of Humanity, consists of a series of foods (fruits, vegetables, legumes, olive oil, wine, fish, and small amounts of meat—preferably white meats) that should be a normal part of nutrition, along with regular physical activity. Consequently, the Mediterranean Diet is not a collection of recipes; it shouldn't be confused with the concept of Italian cooking. It *does*, however, emphasize important human values such as hospitality, neighborliness, intercultural dialogue, and respect for diversity—values which are often expressed in pictures of Italian families enjoying a lively conversation over a plate of pasta and a glass of wine. Several epidemiological studies have demonstrated that the Mediterranean Diet is associated with a lower incidence of mortality from all causes, and it is also related to a lower incidence of cardiovascular disease, type 2 diabetes, and neurodegenerative diseases.

So, what is it that makes the Mamma Mia Diet, itself based on the diets of rural areas of the Mediterranean, possibly be *the* diet of the 21*st* century?

The Mamma Mia Diet (MMD) reflects the changes in the world since the turn of the century. Many people live by themselves and don't really have the time for cooking like our mothers and grandmothers did. The MMD is truly special because is based on the *principles* of the Mediterranean diet, using simple recipes with a modern twist to illustrate how the Mediterranean Diet can reflect a 21st century lifestyle—one where people are have less time to cook, are pressed for time and under a lot of stress, are exposed to more processed food, and do less manual work. We've updated our recipes and cooking techniques to reflect the most recent, scientifically supported nutritional discoveries to make it easy, fast, and modern.

The key words are: **QUALITY, QUANTITY, SYNERGY** and **MODERATION.**

We want people to start thinking differently about food. Food isn't just something that feeds, fuels, and nourishes us; it can be used as medicine for the body, mind, and soul. The Romans said it best long ago: "*Mens sana in corpore sano.*" "Healthy mind in healthy body."

EASY TO FOLLOW, EASY TO LOVE

The MMD is an **easy-to-follow dietary plan** suitable for any age, from childhood though old age.

Here are some simple reasons why the MMD is easy to follow. Remember, the more consistent you are, the better the benefits will be.

Variety and Seasonality

The MMD is based on the **variety** and **seasonality** of plant foods such as fruits, vegetables, legumes and cereals. It also includes a lot of fish and some meat, dairy, olive oil, and even red wine, all in the right proportions. Not to mention, every season you get to enjoy tasty dishes, rich in the best nutrients at their peak of flavor and ripeness.

While most of the ingredients in this book belong to the Mediterranean tradition, a few suggested ingredients come from outside our culinary culture and have been included in the MMD because of their health benefits. These include ginger, turmeric, avocado, and green tea.

All-Inclusive and Complete

There is the right balance to be struck between the macronutrients and micronutrients in one's diet to best support a healthy lifestyle. It is not the effect of any one nutrient that leads to good health, but the **synergy** of different nutrients that leads to improved physical well-being.

The recipes in this book have been selected to create delicious dishes that can help you lose weight, slow down aging, and prevent lifestyle-related diseases. Healthy cooking techniques that reduce the formation of toxic compounds and preserve most of the nutrients have been utilized wherever possible. All good food is included, despite some other diets condemning carbs or animal products. For example, the MMD allows that, every once in a while, there's no harm in indulging in a piece of dark chocolate, a homemade dessert, a slice of pizza, or a scoop of homemade ice cream. In fact, occasional changes to your diet can boost your metabolism and nourish your spirit. The key is **moderation**.

Satiating and Nourishing

The trick to staying full and satisfied after a meal is making sure to eat foods **rich in many nutrients**. The portions given in the MMD may seem conservative (though perhaps not when compared to other diets like Nouvelle Cuisine), but I like to think of them as being "just the right size."

Satiety, the feeling of fullness after eating that suppresses the urge to eat for a period of time after a meal, is beneficial both for losing weight and sticking to a diet. Make sure to eat slowly when possible, as this allows you to feel fuller with less. Italians love to eat in company, and this contributes to our eating less food. This can play an important role in controlling how much you eat and whether you can lose weight.

A New Way of Enjoying Food

The MMD, and Italian-style cuisine in general, is about cultivating conviviality. You can eat healthily while still **enjoying the pleasure of good food** with family and friends. **Conviviality** and the sharing of food are good mechanisms for socialization and improving the health of families and communities, both physical and social.

Grounded and Proven

The recipes in the MMD and the cooking techniques used to make them are scientifically sound and based on the most current nutritional research. Not only that, we've provided you with the **scientific information** to be aware of what is healthy, while giving you the freedom to choose what you prefer to eat according to the season, your tastes, food intolerance/allergies, and lifestyle. Be aware of what your body needs; you **are the "boss" of your health.**

An "Anthropocentric" Diet

The Mamma Mia Diet is an example of an **anthropocentric** meal plan. It focuses on human nature in each of its roles: both the role of the producer, by preferring natural methods and respecting the environment (**sustainability**); and the role of the consumer, the one who eventually eats the food. As defined by the FAO (Food and Agriculture Organization): "Sustainable diets are those diets with low environmental impacts which contribute to food and nutrition security and healthy life for present and future generations."

The MMD encourages you to make positive lifestyle choices, improving your physical and mental health through good nutrition and proper physical activity while remaining respectful of the environment. The MMD should become, at least in part, your new lifestyle—a 21st century lifestyle approach to a healthy and happy life.

Following the Mamma Mia Diet means not only paying attention to what you eat; it also means eating slowly, enjoying food and company, exercising, minimizing physiological stress, drinking in moderation, and not smoking. While the MMD might sound difficult, especially if you have a different lifestyle (such as eating a lot of meat, too few fruits and vegetables, too much junk food, drinking, smoking, and no physical activity), **don't panic**—you can easily get used to this healthy program. Just start at one day a week, and gradually making it your lifestyle. Once you have started adopting better habits, you will find you have no desire to go back to your old ones.

PART I

The Principles of the Mamma Mia! Diet

CHAPTER 1

The Science of the Mamma Mia! Diet

WITH SO MANY DIETS available, it can be tough to figure out which one will actually work best for your needs. To make things harder, dietary guidelines have changed so much over the years as research becomes more accurate in determining what we should eat to achieve optimal health and weight. And knowledge in the field of nutrition is far from complete; no diet can ever be considered "perfect," as individuals will have vastly different needs, capacities, and resources available.

STUDYING THE MEDITERRANEAN DIET

The experimental and epidemiological studies on the health benefits of the Mediterranean diet and the right combination of ingredients in the preparation of traditional Italian recipes are numerous, and have been popular since 1945, when Ancel Keys, a nutritionist who landed in Salerno with the Fifth United States Army, found that the spread of cardiovascular disease in that region of Italy was very limited. Keys and his colleagues proposed that differences in coronary heart disease prevalence among populations were related in some way to physical characteristics and lifestyle—particularly the composition of the diet, especially regarding fat and levels of serum cholesterol. This led to the Seven Countries Study, an enormous project that has influenced and enhanced many studies thereafter, and on which much of the Mamma Mia Diet has been based.

On that subject: only that which can be demonstrated consistently, by rigorous laboratory experiments and long-term epidemiological studies, has scientific value. Consequently, all the information contained in this book is based on reliable scientific data and epidemiological studies published in international, peer-reviewed journals, and conducted by scholars in the field of nutrition and dietetics.

It is recommended, especially for people with preexisting health problems, that you consult your physician before making any changes to your current diet. The literature referred to in this book is reliable, but results are subject to interpretation, and the information presented here may differ from that found in other sources. Always speak to **a qualified nutritionist, dietitian, or physician** before making dramatic changes to your diet.

UNDERSTANDING OBESITY

Obesity is a condition where people accumulate so much body fat that it has a negative effect on their health, leading to several diseases such as type 2 diabetes, cardiovascular disease, respiratory problems (sleep apnea), cancer, depression, and general bad quality of life. The health risks are related to the amount of extra fat accumulated, particularly that stored around the central organs, called **visceral fat**.

How do we know if we are overweight or obese? There are various measures, including checking one's **Body Mass Index (BMI), waist circumference, waist-to-hip ratio, and bio-impedance analysis.**

Body Mass Index (BMI) was a particularly common obesity measurement in the past. BMI is a statistical measurement derived from your height and weight.

To calculate your BMI, plug your weight and height in the following equation: BMI = body weight (kg) / height (m) squared; or, using the imperial system, BMI = body weight (lbs) / height (in) squared x 703. If your BMI is between 25 and 29.9, you are considered overweight. If your BMI is 30 or more, you are considered obese.

Although BMI is considered a useful way to estimate a healthy body *weight*, the problem with BMI is that it does not measure the percentage of body *fat*. BMI measurement can, in fact, be misleading—a muscular person may have a high BMI despite having much less fat than an unfit person, as BMI doesn't take into account the composition of the body—simply weight and height. Luckily, there are other easy tools that may provide a better assessment of body fat, like waist circumference, waist-to-hip ratio, and bio-impedance.

Unlike other measures, **waist circumference** measures visceral fat, the best body part for health indications (though it can be subject to measurement error). A person is considered obese if his/her waist circumference is over 36 inches (90 cm) or 32 inches (80 cm) for males and females, respectively; a waist circumference over 40 inches (100 cm) or 35 inches (88 cm), respectively, predisposes the person to a significant risk of diabetes, heart disease, and stroke.

A similar measure of obesity is the **waist-to-hip ratio,** which examines fat distribution; however, this method is used only infrequently.

Bio-impedance analysis is considered the most accurate test for body fat; however, it is also the least accessible. It measures opposition to a very small electric current as it passes through the body. As lean mass is made up of seventy-three percent water and fat has no water content, this method estimates lean tissue mass (which acts as a conductor) and fat mass (which acts as an insulator) through changes in voltage.

CHAPTER 2

Benefits of the Mamma Mia! Diet

THE WORLD HEALTH ORGANIZATION (WHO) has identified that diet plays an important role in preventing non-communicable diseases, and poor nutrition has become recognized as one of the prime factors responsible for cardiovascular disease, diabetes, malignant cancer, and chronic diseases of the respiratory system (alongside other adverse lifestyle behaviors).

All healthy behaviors are a step in the right direction for improved health and wellness. However, there is so much misleading information in circulation and too many fad diets on the market that finding the right, sustainable balance can be truly challenging!

The Mamma Mia Diet offers everything you need to make the sort of lasting lifestyle choices that lead to healthy weight, increased longevity, overall better health, and higher energy.

Here are several reasons why you should follow the Mamma Mia Diet:

IT'S A LIFESTYLE, NOT A FAD DIET.

Everyone knows there are persons who can eat as much as they want and still not gain weight. At the other extreme are people who seem to gain weight no matter how little they eat.

7

Why? What allows one person to remain at a healthy weight without effort, while another struggles with weight battles?

On a very simple level, weight depends on the number of calories you consume, how many of those calories are stored, and how many are burnt as fuel. Each of these factors is in turn influenced by a combination of genes, diet, and lifestyle. Several diets promise weight loss in no time, but quick weight loss is typically associated with eventual weight gain. Typically, one-third to two-thirds of the weight lost is regained within one year, and almost all is regained within five years. Several long-term studies show that at least one-third of dieters regain more weight than previously lost and suffer more **visceral fat accumulation, changes in adipose tissue composition, insulin resistance,** and **dyslipidemia.**

By choosing to follow the Mamma Mia Diet, you're making a series of healthy lifestyle choices that in the short-term are easy to adopt, yet in the long term, the MMD ensures overall health, and without any extra effort, your weight and figure will take care of themselves. This sounds much better than depriving yourself in the short term just to regain even more weight later, doesn't it? Just pay attention to lifestyle changes, manage your calorie intake through balancing food choices and controlling portions, and meet minimum physical activity requirements. The changes won't be instant, but that's the point—by the time you get to retirement, you'll be thankful that you have constantly maintained a healthy figure, have better bone density, and can look forward to more years of health than your peers.

IT INCREASES LONGEVITY.

About twenty-five percent of variation in human longevity is due to genetic factors identifiable in our DNA sequence (more so in males than females), but environmental factors, which influence nutrition and lifestyle, mediated through epigenetic mechanisms, hold the most responsibility. Recent studies have concluded that both quality and quantity of our diet is linked to aging. Epigenetics, the heritable changes in genetic expression without changing the DNA sequence, is considered to be a major contributor in nutrition-related longevity and the decreased rate of aging.[1] Because diet can influence epigenetic changes, some dietary compounds can be used to treat and even prevent certain diseases.

In recent years, the term *"epigenetic diet"* was coined to refer to the consumption of certain foods, such as soy, grapes, cruciferous vegetables, and green tea, which have been shown to induce epigenetic mechanisms that protect against cancer and aging.[2] These foods, combined with a diet low in protein and sugar, such as the Mamma Mia Diet, allows for the stimulation of the molecular mechanisms which increase lifespan.

Another positive point of the Mediterranean diet's principles is that it can counteract oxidative stress triggered by reactive oxygen species (ROS) via toxic molecules physiologically formed during metabolic reactions. Reactive oxygen species have been proposed as the primary cause of many different degenerative diseases and are known to increase during the aging process. Many studies suggest that they can have both positive and negative roles, depending on the type of reactive oxygen species, when, where and how many are produced. "Good" ROS are those with low reactivity, produced in specific places, at specific times, and in moderate amounts; while "bad" ROS are highly reactive, produced at high concentrations, and are generated continuously and randomly.[3]

A good way to slow the increase of "bad" ROS is by introducing antioxidants, which the MMD is extremely rich in.

In fact, many foods characteristic of the MMD, like fresh fruits, vegetables, nuts, olive oil, and wine, are naturally rich in antioxidative molecules such as vitamins A, C, E, polyphenols, and flavonoids.

---

1 Daniel and Tollefsbol, 2015
2 Hardy and Tollefsbol, 2011
3 Sanz, 2016

The MMD is an eating pattern that can increase not only one's life span, but quality of life, as well!

IT IMPROVES GENERAL HEALTH AND PROVIDES HIGHER ENERGY LEVELS.

Several studies have shown that greater adherence to an eating plan based on a balanced ratio of omega-6 and omega-3 fatty acids, higher amounts of fiber, low amounts of sugar, and the antioxidants and polyphenols found in fruits, vegetables, olive oil, and red wine is associated with a reduction in all-cause mortality, especially heart disease, cancer, diabetes, and depression.

In addition to eating the right food at regular intervals throughout the day, eating this way can jump-start your battery. You will feel more energetic. Slow-burning starches such as whole grain rice and pasta are an important source of energy and nutrients. Sugar and refined flour, by contrast, give you immediate energy, but will be consumed very quickly. You'll find the MMD provides a steady flow of energy that is gradually released throughout the day, without cutting carbohydrates out of your diet. Dehydration can also make you feel tired, so be sure to follow the guidelines for drinking plenty of water during the day. Watch your alcohol intake, as well: alcohol causes dehydration, increases tiredness, and leads to premature aging.

The Mamma Mia Diet also encourages people to spend time in nature, get a good night's sleep, and come together to bond over a home-cooked, healthy meal—all of which are great ways to counteract stress and live a better life. These healthy habits are something we can surely all maintain throughout our life.

CHAPTER 3

Carbohydrates and the Mamma Mia! Diet

IN THE PAST DECADE, carbohydrates (or "carbs") have been harshly criticized, pointed out as *enemy number one* for human health. The reason for this is because they were thought to be the main culprit responsible for obesity, diabetes, and cardiovascular disease.

ARE CARBS REALLY THE ENEMY?

I'm here to tell you, carbs are a *wonderful* thing. Carbs are one of the three essential macronutrients (along with protein and fat). What this means is that these compounds are larger in size compared to micronutrients, and the body needs a relatively large amount of them on a daily basis. Specifically, carbohydrates **provide the energy to move our bodies and the fuel for our organs to function.** Carbohydrates are the *only* source of energy the body uses for our nervous system and red blood cells. For a healthy person, the recommended daily intake of carbs should account for 50–55 percent of their total calorie intake. If we don't eat enough carbs, we don't get the right amount of energy and our body has to get it from somewhere else; for example, by breaking down fat and protein. This can cause many negative side effects such as dizziness, fatigue, headache, and nausea.

Of course, like everything in life, carbs are not perfect. There are good carbs and there are evil ones, so let's try to understand what carbs are, which will be easier to introduce them properly into our everyday diet.

WHAT ARE CARBOHYDRATES?

Carbohydrates are organic compounds present in animal and vegetable food. The name derives from the Greek *carbo* (carbon) and *hydrate* (water). As previously discussed, there are "good" carbs and "bad" carbs. An easy way to identify which is which is by dividing them into two classifications: **simple** and **complex**.

Simple Carbohydrates

Glucose is the most basic and widely found carbohydrate molecule. Fructose and galactose, which are made of just one molecule, are called *monosaccharides* (from the Greek *monos*, meaning single, and *sacchar*, meaning sugar). They are present in different foods and in different quantities (see table below). Sucrose (found in "table sugar" and brown sugar) and lactose (found in dairy products) are disaccharides, meaning they are composed of two monosaccharides. Both disaccharides and monosaccharides are all commonly known as **sugar.**

Many foods, both those occurring in nature and those created by humans, contain simple carbs:

- Fruits, including fresh squeezed fruit juices and vegetables (fructose, glucose)
- Honey (glucose, fructose)
- Milk and dairy products (lactose)
- Candies (glucose)
- Syrups
  - Liquid glucose

- Corn syrup (glucose and fructose)
- Fructose syrup
- Molasses (high in fructose)
- Products with simple sugars (mainly glucose) added:
  - Soft drinks
  - Soda and energy drinks
  - Sauces
  - Cookies, cereals and desserts

SUGAR SUMMARY TABLE

Foods	Monosaccharides		Disaccharides	
	Fructose	Glucose	Lactose	Sucrose
Candies		X		
Fruits, fruit juice, and vegetables	X	X		
Honey and maple syrup	X	X		
White and brown sugar				X
Milk and dairy products			X	
Syrups	X	X		
Soft drinks, sport drinks, energy drinks, sauces, cookies, cereals, and desserts		X		

Is Sugar a Killer?

As in all things, quantity and quality are the keys. Sugar adds a sweet taste to food and, most of the time, is associated with a positive feeling, which is why it is added to so many foods.

As Paracelsus said, "It is the dose that makes the poison." *Small* doses of sugar will not kill you. The World Health Organization guidelines recommend that sugar intake should not exceed ten percent of your total daily calories, and should be limited to about five percent for additional health benefits. For example, in a diet of 1,500 calories per day, the amount of sugar should not exceed 7.5 teaspoons (37.5 g), or about 150 calories. For context, a small glass of soda contains about 6 teaspoons (30 g) of sugar, which is roughly equivalent to one daily dose of sugar for someone on a 1,500 calorie diet.

Simple sugar is digested quickly, causing an immediate spike in blood sugar. This causes a release of insulin (the hormone that controls blood sugar levels), allowing sugar to enter cells to be used as energy or be transformed and stored as fat. The blood sugar level then decreases. These quick increases and decreases in insulin secretion trigger our brain to want more, leading to cravings. In this way, sugar sets up an extremely powerful drive to make us eat more, burn less energy, and gain weight.

In the past century, the food industry has started adding increasing amounts of sugar to make their foods and beverages as attractive as possible, precisely because our brain likes that flavor. Soon, we became addicted to it. This is mainly due to the consumption of sucrose and high-fructose corn syrup (HFCS) present in industrial foods and beverages in the United States. A growing body of scientific evidence is showing that fructose can trigger processes that lead to liver toxicity and non-communicable diseases (NCD) such as atherosclerosis, type 2 diabetes, and obesity.[1]

In Italy, fructose is rarely used as a sweetener in processed foods; instead, sucrose is added. Data from the relevant scientific literature indicates that normal consumption of fructose (approximately 10–12 teaspoons (50–60 g) per day) does not increase the risk of atherosclerosis, type 2 diabetes, or obesity any more than the consumption of other sugars. Conversely, a high intake of fructose combined with

1 Lustig, 2010

a high energy intake (through high consumption of carbs) may have negative health effects.[2]

I CAN'T GIVE UP SWEETS … WHICH SIMPLE SUGAR SHOULD I CHOOSE?

Fruits, honey, and maple syrup are all better choices than refined sugar because they contain vitamins and minerals. Still, your intake should not exceed the maximum daily recommended dose of 5–10 percent of your total calories. If you crave something sweet, fruit is by far the best choice, as it is rich in vitamins, minerals, antioxidants, and fiber which counter the sugar spike in the blood. Personally, I'll eat an apple and feel satisfied. Apples also contain pectin, **a type of dietary fiber that makes you feel fuller for longer.** This high concentration of pectin contributes to the relatively low Glycemic Index (GI) of apples.

In terms of sweeteners, **stevia** is natural, made from a leaf related to popular garden flowers like asters and chrysanthemums. In South America and Asia, people have been using stevia leaves to sweeten drinks like tea for many years.

However, stevia available commercially gets so significantly refined that the FDA finds it hard to label stevia products. Instead, it labels highly processed types of stevia as **novel sweeteners**. Novel sweeteners are combinations of various types of sweeteners, which I would recommend you use only with caution. The European Food Safety Authority (EFSA) recommends a dosage of 1.9–2.3 mg per kg of weight daily.

---

2 Kolderup and Svihus, 2015

Artificial Sweeteners

Often, people ask the question, "Are artificial sweeteners better than simple sugars?"

The answer is not at all, for two reasons. First, even though you reduce the number of calories you're taking in, you aren't reducing the sweet taste. Consuming artificial sweeteners gives a different signal to the brain, but we still crave something sweet. It still triggers the vicious circle of consumption/false satiety/serotonin/craving. Second, artificial sweeteners are chemical compounds (such as saccharin, aspartame, and acesulfame) that are possibly responsible for different side effects, although there are no conclusive studies at the moment. Only time will tell us, but in the meantime, I would prefer to be on the safer side of the fence.

Safe, Sweet Treats

The safest way to indulge your sweet tooth is in moderation. Once in a while—for example, on the weekends or at the restaurant—we can enjoy something sweet as a treat. A dessert after a meal will not kill you, and actually is considered better than a snack, because the sugar will be mixed with other ingredients and will be absorbed more slowly, reducing the sugar spike. However, if you want **to lose weight,** I would recommend limiting your consumption of sweets to **"very rarely."**

Gelato, a staple of Italian cuisine and well-known to lovers of Italy around the world, is a great choice when looking for a sweet treat after a meal or on a special occasion. If you are going to go for a *gelato,* look for homemade Italian-style brands made with simple and genuine ingredients: milk, cream, eggs, sugar, and vanilla. *Gelato* is caloric, so if you are trying to reduce the number of calories, opt for **small sizes (half a cup)** or share with a friend! If you absolutely must have a topping, it is best to choose fresh berries.

And what about chocolate? The so-called "natural drug," chocolate is definitely one of life's little pleasures which is difficult to resist. Chocolate is rich in calories—500 calories per 3.5 oz (100 g) for **dark chocolate** and 600 calories per 3.5 oz or 100 g for milk chocolate—but **in moderation** it can be part of our diet. Make allowances for it in your daily calorie intake. I recommend a dose of dark chocolate, 1 oz or about 30 g, two or three times a week. Dark chocolate (at least 70% cocoa) is certainly the best choice because it is almost sugar-free and is rich in many nutrients (such as antioxidants, flavonoids, and minerals). It also contains caffeine and theobromine, which are both involved in energy metabolism, adiposity, and obesity,[3] and cathechins, which are compounds that may help prevent cancers and heart diseases.

Getting Over Sugar Addiction

We crave sugar not because we need it, but because our palate has been altered by abusing it too much. The key is to re-train our palate to prefer less sugar. This is the only way to beat temptation for good!

Seven simple rules will help you say no to sugar. Your waistline will thank you!

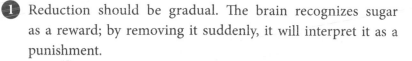

1. Reduction should be gradual. The brain recognizes sugar as a reward; by removing it suddenly, it will interpret it as a punishment.

2. Gradually get used to taking your beverages unsweetened, including coffee, tea, and milk. A few years ago, I started reducing the amount of sugar in my espresso and cappuccino each day. After just a few weeks, I could not drink them sweet

3 Huang et al., 2016

anymore. My palate refused that taste and now loves the real coffee aroma. Do not try to replace sugar with other sweeteners (natural or artificial); you might reduce the number of calories, but the sweet taste will remain, meaning you will still desire the sugar.

3 Avoid soda, which are rich in empty calories and lack nutrients, and pre-packaged fruit juices (which are packed with sugar unless "without sugar added" is indicated on the label).

4 Limit the amount of processed sweets such as cookies, snacks, candies, ice cream, and spreads. Watch out for "light" products; to compensate for the lack of sugar, more fat is added to enrich the flavor of these foods. The terms "light" and "diet" are not regulated by any standards, so "light" could indicate less weight and "diet" can be placed on any product, healthy or not.

5 Eat unsweetened cereals; for example, oats, which are high in fiber and encourage good intestinal flora.

6 Try to make your desserts at home from fresh ingredients, and limit the amount of sugar you use. Replace sugar with apple-sauce or grape juice.

7 Learn to satisfy your sweet cravings with a piece of fresh fruit, two or three nuts, or a small handful of dried fruits. (When buying dried fruits, make sure to read the labels; some products have sugar added).

In no time, your palate will get used to the different taste (it takes about two months for our body to adjust to a new behavior), and your health and weight will benefit from it.

COMPLEX CARBOHYDRATES

Complex carbs are long chains of monosaccharide sugars, and are therefore called polysaccharides (*poly*, meaning many). Depending on the number and the type of monosaccharides they contain, they perform different functions. Complex carbs take longer to break down and give a more sustained level of energy in comparison to simple carbs. Whole grain carbs are even better, because they contain more fiber and nutrients.

Starch, one of the main forms of complex carbs, originates from the structural components of plants such as potatoes, rice, wheat, and corn. It is an insoluble fiber, which means it does not dissolve in the gut, but instead keeps its form rather well and collects waste on its way through the body.

Other complex carbs exist which are more soluble, such as pectin (found in fruits and vegetable peels) and those found in the softer parts of fruits and vegetables. These ferment our food, which assists with satiety, protects against type 2 diabetes and heart disease, and keeps us regular, all while assisting weight loss.

Whole Grain Carbohydrates

You almost certainly will have heard that whole grains are healthy and make a good ally in losing weight.

But what *are* whole grains?

Grains are the seeds of cereal crops such as wheat, rye, rice, oat and barley. They are comprised of three edible parts—the bran, the germ, and the endosperm. In whole grains, all these components are present, whereas refined white flour consists mainly of the starchy endosperm, without the bran and germ. Refined white flour became popular because it produced baked goods with a softer taste, but the bran and germ both contain important nutrients (protein, minerals, healthy fats, B vitamins, antioxidants, and fiber) which are lost when grain is refined.

Since 2000, recommendations for whole grain intake have been included in the Dietary Guidelines for Americans: "Eat at least 3 oz (80 g) or equivalent of whole grain daily, and at least half of all grains consumed should be whole grain."[4] The National Health and Nutrition Examination Survey in the United States also suggests that greater whole grain consumption is associated with better micronutrient intakes and healthier body weight in children and adults.[5]

Whole grains offer the following benefits:

1. They are high in fiber, helping to maintain a healthy intestinal tract.

2. They are slow to digest due to their medium Glycemic Index (GI), which helps regulate blood sugar.

3. They are loaded with vitamins and minerals, improving nutrient density.

4. They are satisfying, helping control appetite.

In terms of the Mamma Mia Diet, a recent systematic study indicated that reducing white bread consumption (but not whole grain bread consumption) within a Mediterranean-style food diet is associated with lower weight gain and abdominal fat.[6] It is important to note: **food made with white flour mixed with bran is not whole grains**. In fact, according to the definition of the Whole Grains Council, "Whole grains or foods made from them must contain all the essential parts and naturally-occurring nutrients of the entire grain seed in their original proportions. If grain has been processed, the food product should deliver the same rich balance of nutrients that are found in the original grain seed."

---

4 USDA, Dietary Guidelines for Americans: 6*th*, 2015, USDA. Dietary Guidelines for Americans: 7*th*, 2015.

5 Albertson et al., 2016

6 Serra-Majem and Bautista-Castano, 2015

Wheat Grain and Gluten Intolerance

Wheat grain has been altered by the food industry to provide crops that are more resistant to drought and bake more easily. Some studies show that the older grains tend to have lower levels of gliadins, a type of peptides which, along with glutenins, when in the presence of water, form **gluten**.

In modern grains, the quantity of gluten is higher than in older grains, and that seems to cause most sensitivities in people diagnosed with **gluten intolerance**. Our intestines have not fully adapted to these changes.

In addition, we are eating more wheat products now than ever before. Think about all those fast food meals, with rich sandwiches made using poor quality bread. My recommendation is to use "old" grain products as much as possible, and alternate with gluten-free grains such as rice, quinoa, corn, millet, and buckwheat. Remember: a varied diet is always the most complete one. In the recipe section of this book, I've tried to include dishes prepared with different types of cereals, because each one has a different nutritional profile. **Variety** is one of the main principles of the MMD.

Note: Many people perceive benefits from a gluten-free diet without a clear scientific explanation. There is no evidence that processed gluten-free foods are "healthier" than their gluten-containing counterparts. If there is no medical evidence of celiac disease, it is useless to follow a gluten-free diet. In fact, it has been shown that overweight, new-onset insulin resistance and deficiencies in B vitamins, folate, and iron, are actually consequences of a gluten-free diet.[7]

---

7 Reilly, 2016

GLYCEMIC INDEX (GI)

We've mentioned it a few times, but what exactly is meant by a food's Glycemic Index?

The **Glycemic Index (GI)** is a value assigned to carbohydrates based on how slowly or quickly they cause an increase of glucose levels in the blood. The Glycemic Index uses a scale ranging from 0 to 100, in which pure glucose serves as a reference point (GI = 100).

All foods can be distributed into three groups[8]:

- High GI: 70 or more
- Medium GI: between 55 and 70
- Low GI: less than 55.

---

8 A complete GI table for more than 1,000 foods can be found in the article "International tables of Glycemic Index and glycemic load values" Atkinson et al., 2008.

Classification	GI Range	Example
High GI	> 70	Glucose (grape sugar), high fructose corn syrup, white bread, most white rice (only rice endosperm), cornflakes (Kellog's), extruded breakfast cereals, maltose, sweet potato (70), white potato (83), date palm.
Medium GI	55-70	White sugar or sucrose, whole bread, pasta, pita bread, basmati rice, unpeeled boiled potato, grape juice, raisins, prunes, pumpernickel bread, regular ice cream, banana, lychee, pineapple.
Low GI	< 55	Fructose, beans (black, pinto, kidney, lentil, peanut, chickpea), small seeds (sunflower, flax, pumpkin, poppy, sesame, hemp), walnuts, cashews, most whole intact grains (durum, spelt, kamut wheat, millet, oat, rye, rice, barley), whole meal spaghetti, most vegetables, most sweet fruits (peaches, strawberries, mangoes), tagatose, mushrooms, chilis

Carbohydrates with a low GI value (55 or less) are more slowly digested, absorbed and metabolized, and cause a lower and slower rise in blood glucose and, therefore, insulin secretion.

Several recent scientific studies have shown that individuals who follow a low-GI diet over many years are at a significantly lower risk for developing both type 2 diabetes and cardiovascular disease.[9] High blood glucose levels or repeated glycemic "spikes" following a meal can promote these diseases by increasing systemic glycated stress, oxidative stress to one's cardiovascular system, and a direct increase in insulin levels.[10]

A practical limitation of the GI is that it does not measure insulin production due to rises in blood sugar; it simply measures a rise in blood sugar. As a result, two foods could have the same GI but produce different amounts of insulin, and therefore have different health properties. There's also some argument regarding reference points; for example, white bread is sometimes used as a reference food, resulting in a different set of GI values for all foods (if white bread has a GI of 100, then glucose would have a GI of about 140). Other things that can affect a food's GI value include ripeness (in the case of fruits like bananas) and differences in how the food was prepared.

To give an example (and because it plays a starring role in many MMD recipes), the GI of pasta is very different for pasta that is cooked "*al dente*" or for a longer time. Pasta "*al dente*" has a lower GI than overcooked pasta because the cooking process makes the starch more easily available to enzymes that hydrolyze the starch (in a process called gelatinization, which ultimately increases blood sugar).

The GI value of food may also change when eaten with other foods: for example, the GI value of pasta and rice decreases when they are eaten with fiber-rich vegetables and olive oil. Thankfully, there are many delicious recipes in the Italian culinary repertoire that pair pasta and vegetables together! (This is another reason why it is a healthy habit to start your meal with a salad—it decreases the GI of the following dishes).

---

9 *Chiu et al., 2011*
10 Temelkova-Kurktschiev et al., 2000

Last but not least, the rate at which individuals digest carbohydrates also varies, so there will be some individual differences in GI values from person to person.

Carbs and Weight Loss: Debunking the Myths So, in order to lose weight, should we avoid carbs?

Not at all! In fact, good carbs can *help* us lose weight. Carbs are not something to be feared and avoided; everything depends on the type of carbs, the amount, the preparation method, and the time we eat them during the day. Several studies have demonstrated that the Italian diet is one of the healthiest diets in the world, and Italian cuisine is full of carb-rich foods. After all, could you imagine asking an Italian to go without pasta?

Carbs make us feel happy and satisfied; they are one of life's pleasures. Think about a plate of **pasta**, for example. Pasta is one of the most popular comfort foods in the world; we Italians certainly cannot live without it. We are a nation of pasta lovers, after all, and pasta gives you so many options on top of being an economic food for the whole family. Several studies have even shown that **whole grain pasta** is a good ally **in losing weight**. That may be surprising, but it's true! So if you have banished pasta from your cupboards in an effort to squeeze into your old jeans, you've made a big mistake.

And while we're on the topic, there's no reason to be afraid of **bread.** Bread is a staple in the Italian diet and is considered the **food of human civilization**—a symbol of plenty, even a religious symbol. Many anthropologists have observed that smell of fresh bread is nearly universally recognized as something good, which is impossible to give up. I still remember the smell of the fresh homemade **whole grain bread** I used to make with my grandmother when I was a child. My favorite part was kneading the dough.

Many people substitute bread with crackers and breadsticks, thinking they are less caloric. This is a myth: they are *more* caloric and contain unhealthy fats. When you buy bread, try to purchase **fresh whole grain bread** and keep away from bread containing dough conditioners, preservatives, GMOs, added sugar, and artificial flavors and coloring (though the best bread remains the one prepared by my grandmother, using only simple and nutritious ingredients; refer to page 178 for her recipe!) Finally, **never combine bread with other complex carbs** (such as pasta and rice) in one meal. Not only are you adding too many carbs to your meal, you're not following the Italian rules!

WHAT ABOUT PIZZA?

Pizza is a food that holds a special place in pretty much everyone's hungry heart. Nobody can say no to pizza, from adults to kids; it unites omnivores, vegetarians, and vegans alike.

Eating pizza is a pleasure of life that we *can* indulge in, but *how* we eat it makes all the difference.

Enjoy pizza (though not more than once a week as a main course) **the Italian way**: a thin crust (better if prepared with whole grain flour) with fresh tomato sauce, olive oil (extra virgin), mozzarella cheese (a reasonable amount), and only one or two other healthy toppings (vegetables are best). Clearly, this is better than thick slices overloaded with huge amounts of cheese and unhealthy toppings that make pizza very salty on top of being a caloric juggernaut. If your pizza is prepared with regular flour, start your meal with a plate of simple salad (for example, lettuce, cucumber, and tomato dressed with olive oil and lemon juice or balsamic vinegar) because the fiber contained in these vegetable will positively affect your glucose absorption.

DO's and DON'Ts

If you're having trouble getting the right daily dose of good carbs, I've summarized things and put together a few DO's and DON'Ts/ LIMITs to make things easier.

DO's

1. **DO** eat whole grain varieties. For example, 1 serving of pasta (about 2.5 oz or 70 g), 1–2 servings of bread (1–2 slices, 1 oz or 28 g per serving), or, once in while, a slice of pizza (Italian style!). Pasta, when you eat it, should be the main food of your meal, and not a side dish. Some days you can substitute pasta with about 1 serving (scarce ½ cup or about 70 g) of rice, spelt, barley, or other grains. The amount in grams may slightly vary for each different type of grain.
2. **DO** eat pasta and other grains with vegetables.
3. **DO** eat pasta with (a little) sauce; remember: it's pasta with sauce, not sauce with pasta!
4. **DO** eat variety of fresh seasonal fruits.
5. **DO** eat dark chocolate (1 oz or about 30 g, about 2 two small squares, 150 kilocalories, 2–3 times a week).

DON'Ts/LIMITS

1. **DON'T** eat pasta, rice, or other grains with bread.
2. **DON'T** eat processed foods; for example, crackers, cookies, snacks, sweetened cereal.
3. **DON'T** eat fast food or foods rich in sugar or drink carbonated drinks.

4. **DON'T** overload (or at least **LIMIT**) potatoes and sugar and choose fruits, honey, and maple syrup where possible.

5. **DON'T** add sweeteners to your coffee and drinks.

6. **LIMIT** cakes, *gelato,* and sweets. Ideally, make your own ones at home and add less sugar.

Carbohydrates and the Mamma Mia Diet: A Summary

Why should we eat carbs?
Because they are the main **source of energy** for our bodies, like fuel for our car. During their metabolism, carbohydrates provide 4 calories/gram.

What carbs should we eat and how much?
Carbs should make up **50–55 percent of our caloric intake,** with **sugar making up no more of 10 percent** (or 5 percent, if possible) of our daily caloric intake.

Complex carbs are the key, with whole grain varieties being the obvious choice, as they contain more nutrients). **Daily intake should be 5–7 oz or 140–200 g/ day,** depending on age, gender, and physical activity. **You should also aim for 1 oz or about 25–30 g of fiber per day**.

When during the day should we eat carbs?
It is better to eat carbs for **breakfast and lunch,** because it is the time of the day when our bodies need more energy.

CHAPTER 4

Fruits and Vegetables and the Mamma Mia! Diet

To LIVE A HEALTHY and long life, fruits and vegetables need to be at the heart of our diet. Personally, I love them; I cannot live without these **natural friends**. When I was a little girl, I spent summers at my grandparents' country house, and I still remember eating whatever nature offered during that season: delicious tomatoes, eggplant, and zucchini and wonderful peaches, watermelons, and apricots. Today, living in the town center, the only way to get fresh, local, and seasonal fruits and vegetables is to purchase them at my local market. Wherever you live, I recommend you visit your closest market for your fresh produce!

WHAT BENEFITS DO FRUITS AND VEGETABLES PROVIDE?

Eating a lot of fruits and vegetables is essential, both for good health and weight control. Most **fruits and vegetables** are **low in calories, low in fat, and have no cholesterol; instead, they are high in fiber and water,** essential ingredients for successful weight

31

control. They also contain plenty of **micronutrients** like **vitamins,
minerals,** and **bioactive compounds,** and **fiber, water, and antioxidants,** all of which are important for helping us look good, feel
our best, and protect ourselves from disease. So enjoy a wide variety of fruits and vegetables every day. They're like a concentrated
health cocktail.

I won't go into detail about the names and functions of each
and every micronutrient; that's a book unto itself, and would detract
from the purpose of this book. However, we will briefly summarize
the types of micronutrients here, with a brief explanation of their
benefits.

Suffice it to say that a practical and achievable way of ensuring correct micronutrient consumption is to consume as wide a variety of
fresh produce, grains, dairy, and protein as possible:

- **Fiber,** in addition to keeping the gut "clean" and helping you
  achieve a flat stomach, also promotes satiety and reduces
  the risk of lifestyle-related diseases, including diabetes and
  heart disease. For more information on the role of fiber in
  the human body, see Chapter 3.
- **Vitamins** are organic compounds which are needed (in
  small quantities) to **sustain life.** We obtain vitamins from
  food because the human body either **does not produce
  them or produces insufficient quantities.** There are thir-
  teen different vitamins, each of which have different and
  highly varied functions at the cellular level. Some vitamins
  affect cell division, others govern synthesis of our DNA,
  maintenance of vision, metabolism of carbohydrates ... the
  list goes on. Consuming insufficient quantities of vitamins
  means the most vital actions of the body cannot be performed. No matter how much time we spend at the gym or
  dieting, we can't consider ourselves healthy unless we first
  function well.

- **Minerals**, even trace minerals, are also critical for the proper functioning of the body. We get them from the food we eat and the water we drink. Most minerals aid metabolism, water balance, and bone health, but they also participate in hundreds of other small ways to effectively **boost health**.
- **Bioactive compounds** include polyphenols, flavonoids, and anthocyanins. These substances have antioxidant and anti-inflammatory properties.
- **Water** helps remove excess liquid and toxins from the body.

HOW MUCH FRUITS AND VEGETABLES SHOULD I EAT?

The health benefits of fruits and vegetables are thought to derive from a combination of all these components. You will almost certainly have heard about **nutrient density.** This refers to the quantity of micronutrients contained in a certain volume of food. Foods that are rich in nutrients and low in calories are considered **nutrient-dense**, while foods rich in calories and low in nutrients are considered **nutrient-poor**. To give you a simple example, **fruits and vegetables** are nutrient-dense, while cookies and fries contain very few micronutrients by comparison, and so are nutrient-poor.

We should aim to consume at least two servings of fruits and three servings of vegetables every day. I personally consume more of both; however, everyone—including adults, children, and elderly people—should add fruits and vegetables to every meal. In this way, you can be certain to consume a good supply of fiber, vitamins, and minerals. A single serving of fruits is **4–5 oz (or 110–140 g);** for example, a medium-sized piece of fruit like an apple, a pear, or an orange, or two small fruits, such as plums or apricots.

Regarding **vegetables,** we should distinguish between cooked and raw. If consuming **raw**, the serving size is **2–2.5 oz (or 60–70 g);** if we **cook them**, the weight *before* cooking should be **9 oz (or about 250 g),** as vegetables lose nutrients as they lose their water weight.

WHAT FRUITS AND VEGETABLES SHOULD I EAT?

The 2015–2020 Dietary Guidelines for Americans (DGA) promote the inclusion of a variety of vegetables from all five of the following subgroups: dark green, red and orange, legumes (beans and peas), starchy, and other groups of the rainbow.[1] Numerous observational epidemiological studies have shown an inverse relationship between the consumption of fruits, vegetables, and legumes and the prevalence of cancer and cardiovascular disease risk factors, including obesity, hypertension, and type 2 diabetes.

In fact, it was estimated in one study that 35 percent of cancers could be attributed to diet and that dietary modification is a valid strategy for cancer prevention. The World Cancer Research Fund and the American Institute for Cancer Research are responsible for producing recommendations for cancer prevention, and one recommendation given asks people to **"eat mostly foods of plant origin."** The consumption of 5–6 portions of fruits and vegetables a day is associated with reduced cancer risk and improved survival after cancer diagnosis.

The scientific studies relating to dietary influence over cancer can be challenging to interpret, especially because food and eating patterns are inherently complex and multifactorial. A diet high in fruits and vegetables provides numerous micronutrients such as folate, polyphenol, carotenoids, and fiber, and focusing on a specific nutrient might result in misleading findings. Consequently, new research has instead suggested that analyses of dietary patterns are a more useful strategy for cancer prevention.[2]

Therefore, **adherence to the Mediterranean lifestyle**, with the right *equilibrium* of different foods, high consumption of fruits and

---

1 U.S. Department of Health and Human Services and U.S. Department of Agriculture. 2015–2020

2 Mayne et al., 2016

vegetables, dietary fiber, and probiotic products, maintenance of a healthy body weight, and participation in regular physical exercise is **effective for cancer prevention.**

FRESH VS FROZEN

The eternal question of those with busy schedules: should we eat fresh or frozen fruits and vegetables?

The fact is that **freezing can slightly alter the nutritional composition** of fruits and vegetables however, this is sometimes to the *benefit* of the frozen product. For example, freezing leafy green vegetables like spinach decreases the amount of folate, while vitamin K is not affected; however, by the time fresh spinach reaches our plate, it's likely that several days have already passed and decomposition has begun, resulting in nutrient loss. Consequently, sometimes the choice is in favor of the frozen product and sometimes in favor of the fresh one.

It all depends on the freezing process used. Fruits and vegetables that are to be frozen are generally picked at their peak ripeness, when they are the most nutritious. Vegetables are often harvested, washed, blanched, cut, frozen, and packaged within a few hours. Fruits tend not to undergo blanching, as this can greatly affect their texture; instead they are treated with vitamin C to preserve color, and sugar is may be added to increase sweetness. (Read labels carefully to find out if any additives have been added.)

Results from several studies show that the nutrient content of frozen and fresh goods vary slightly, although differences in processing and measuring methods can influence results. We can say that, in general, freezing can preserve some nutrients, but freshly picked fruits and vegetables straight from the farm or your own garden are of the highest quality. However, when you do not have time to clean and prepare vegetables, frozen is better than not eating any at all! **Choose a mix of fresh and frozen products to ensure you get the best range of nutrients possible.** I personally sometimes buy frozen peas, whose nutritional value is similar to fresh ones; however, the taste of fresh peas is certainly better. I always prefer to buy fresh fruit because eating fresh fruit is a pleasure for all senses that the frozen alternative does not offer.

EAT THE RAINBOW

There is no single fruit or vegetable that is the elixir of long life, but each of them provides us with different nutrients. Fruits and vegetables come in all kind of shapes, sizes, colors, flavors, and textures. With each season, nature offers us a wide variety of each to choose from. Regardless of your preferences, following the **rule of the rainbow will give you the best variety of nutrients**.

Variety is the key. The term "eat the rainbow" is a simplified way of saying that fruits and vegetables aren't created equally and that the color of foods can tell us a lot about their nutritional value. Eating a variety of colors is one sure method to get as many different vitamins, minerals, and nutrients as possible. Plants often derive their colors from the various phytochemicals they contain. These substances offer us different nutrients when consumed.

In order to eat the rainbow, you should try to consume red, orange and yellow, green, blue, purple, and white foods throughout the seasons. The recipes in this book represent my contribution to helping people eat the rainbow!

Red: The Color of Passion

The red hue in foods is due to natural pigments called anthocyanins and lycopenes.

Anthocyanins have excellent free-radical scavenging and anti-oxidant properties, and they protect our body's cells from damage. They are found in pomegranates, raspberries, red grapes (and red wine), strawberries, beets, red bell peppers, red cabbages, and red onions.

Lycopenes have been studied for their antioxidant properties and are considered very good antioxidants. Several studies suggest a link between lycopene consumption and prostate and gastrointestinal cancer prevention.[3] They are better absorbed when cooked and, because they are fat-soluble, consumption with oil increases absorption and improves passage between the digestive tract and blood stream. Lycopenes are found in foods such as cherries, papaya, pink grapefruit, watermelon, and tomatoes. Adding extra virgin olive oil to a tomato dish is an excellent way of maximizing the benefits from lycopenes in tomatoes. The Italian *"passata di Pomodoro,"* a tomato sauce for pasta, is a staple of Italian cuisine which allows us to get plenty of lycopenes.

Orange and Yellow: The Colors of Friendship

Orange and yellow fruits and vegetables owe their beautiful color to natural pigments called **carotenoids**. Carotenoids also act as

3 Kim and Kim 2015; Martí et al., 2016

antioxidants. They have strong cancer-fighting properties, anti-inflammatory and immune system benefits, and are sometimes associated with cardiovascular disease prevention. There are more than 600 types of carotenoids. The most common ones in the Western diet, and the most studied, are alpha-carotene, beta-carotene, beta-cryptoxanthin, lutein, zeaxanthin, and lycopenes.

Nutritionally, there is another, potentially more useful grouping of carotenoids: provitamin A and non-provitamin A. **Provitamin A carotenoids** can be turned into **vitamin A (retinol)** in the intestine or liver. Vitamin A is an important component of human health, as it helps maintain **healthy eyes, healthy mucus membranes, and good immunity**. You may have heard that eating carrots is good for your eyes, or that eating carrots helps you see in the dark; this is true, to a point, as they contain carotenoids. Alpha-carotene, beta-carotene, and beta-cryptoxanthin are provitamin A carotenoids; lutein, zeaxanthin, and lycopene are not. Carotenoids like lycopenes are better absorbed when lightly cooked compared to when they're eaten raw. They are found in different yellow/orange fruits and vegetables such as apricots, mango, oranges, peaches, pineapple, tangerines, carrots, corn, kale, spinach, squash, and sweet potatoes.

Green: The Color of Energy

It is no surprise that green foods are packed with a lot of nutrients. Go for green to get **antioxidants** such as **carotenoids** and **flavonoids**, and other nutrients including **chlorophyll** and **folate**. Folate is a B vitamin that helps with the formation of red and white blood cells and aids in all kinds of cell divisions. The nutrients present in green food have been found to lower the risk of cancer, blood pressure, and LDL cholesterol levels, as well as maintain retinal (eye) health and boost immunity. Green fruits and vegetables contain lots of **fiber, which helps digestion and weight control.** Green vegetables are also a good source of **calcium,** which is a mineral essential for healthy bones and teeth. Green fruits include green tomatoes, avocado, kiwi, green grapes, green apples, and lime. When it comes to green vegetables, there are many options. Choose from artichokes, arugula (rocket), asparagus, broccoli, celery, green beans, kale, peas, spinach, and all dark, leafy greens.

Blue and Purple: The Colors of Peace

The power of purple goes beyond its vibrant color, and often indicates high nutrient density and antioxidant levels. Similar to orange and yellow foods, **anthocyanins** contribute to this beautiful color, which have shown to fight cancer, inflammation, and aging due to their **antioxidant properties**. Each season, you can enjoy purple fruits and vegetables such as blackberries, blueberries, purple figs (my favorite), purple grapes (like strawberry grapes), raisins, eggplants, and purple cabbage.

White: The Color of Purity

White fruits and vegetables contain plenty of nutrients, including **anthocyanins,** which help lower cholesterol and blood pressure; **sulfur,** which detoxifies the liver and helps with protein structure and skin health; **allicin,** which is found in garlic and has anti-cancer properties; and **quercetin,** which has anti-inflammatory properties. White foods also boost immunity and help avoid weight gain. The only white foods people should avoid are processed, refined ones, such as those produced using a lot of processed white sugar or refined white flour. Healthy white foods include those which are tan or brown on the outside and white inside, such as **pears.** Other important white foods include apples, bananas, white grapes, cauliflower, cabbage, fennel, garlic, ginger, mushrooms, onions, potatoes, and white corn.

CITRUS FRUITS

Citrus fruits (including lemons, oranges, mandarins, clementines, and grapefruits) deserve a special mention. These are staples in the Italian diet and my favorite winter fruits. They have a high concentration of many nutrients and contain high amounts of **pectin**, a soluble dietary fiber which transports cholesterol and binds to carbohydrates in the gut, slowing glucose absorption. Citrus fruits are linked to cholesterol and diabetes control for this reason.

Citrus fruits are also a very important source of **vitamin C**, a critical water-soluble vitamin. We are unable to synthesize vitamin C ourselves, so all of our requirements must be obtained from food. Vitamin C is required for the **biosynthesis of collagen, L-carnitine, and certain neurotransmitters**. Collagen is an essential component of connective tissue, which plays a vital role in wound healing. Vitamin C is also involved in **protein metabolism** and is an important **physiological antioxidant** which has been shown to regenerate other antioxidants within the body, including alpha-tocopherol (vitamin E). By limiting the damaging effects of free radicals through antioxidant activity, vitamin C can help prevent or delay the development of certain cancers, cardiovascular disease, and other diseases caused by oxidative stress.

It has been shown that the antioxidant properties of vitamin C are much higher when ingested in the form of food rather than with supplements. Fruits and vegetables that are good sources of vitamin C include kiwi, strawberries, broccoli, Brussels sprouts, red and green peppers, and tomatoes. The vitamin C content of food may be reduced by prolonged storage or by cooking, because vitamin C is a water-soluble vitamin destroyed easily by heat (though steaming or micro-waving may lessen cooking losses). Fortunately, many of the best food sources of vitamin C, such as fruits and vegetables, can be consumed raw. Consuming 2–3 servings a day of fruits and vegetables can pro-vide 70–90 mg of vitamin C, the necessary amount for proper functioning.

LEGUMES: "THE POOR MAN'S MEAT"

Legume is a general term used to describe the seeds of plants from the legume family *Papilionaceous* and includes lentils, peas, chick-peas, beans, soybeans, and peanuts.

The use of legumes as food dates back to more than 20,000 years ago in Asian cultures, while common beans were grown for the first time by people in Mexico and Peru 5,000 years ago. Legumes have been an important part of the diets of many cultures associated with long lifespan, such as the Japanese, who regularly eat soy foods and their derivatives, and Mediterranean cultures, where lentils, chick-peas, and white beans are normally present in traditional dishes (refer to Part III: Recipes and Seasonal Menus for some examples).

Legumes have long been considered **a particularly economical dietary source of protein** and are higher in protein than most other plant foods. It is for this reason that the 68th United Nations General Assembly declared 2016 the International Year of Legumes.

The **nutritional profile of legumes** is particularly remarkable: they are a rich source of **vegetable protein (about 20 percent) with good digestibility.** With the exception of soybeans, which are rich in polyunsaturated fatty acids (PUFAs), legumes are low in fat, are a good source of folate, vitamins B6 and B1, iron, and potassium, and contain low glycemic index carbohydrates. In addition, legumes are particularly **rich in healthy fiber** like **resistant starch** and **raffinose**. These types of fiber pass through the digestive tract undigested and, once in the colon, act as "prebiotics" or "food" for the beneficial bacteria residing there. Legumes also contain several phenolic compounds, which may protect against some cancers.

The "dark side" of legumes is the presence of certain anti-nutritional factors like phytic acid, which inhibit digestion and the absorption of some nutrients such as iron, zinc, and, to a lesser extent, calcium. (This is why legumes should not be eaten raw!)

Many epidemiological studies have confirmed that eating legumes can extend one's life by preventing chronic disease, including cardiovascular disease, diabetes, cancer, and obesity.[4] A recent study demonstrated that consumption of 2⅔ cups (400 g) of fresh legumes a week decreases the events of ischemic heart diseases.[5]

However, despite American guidelines suggesting 1½ cups (225 g) of fresh legumes or ½ cup (100 g) a week in dry weight, the USDA Economic Research Service estimates that only fourteen percent of Americans consume dried beans. Meanwhile, the most recent Italian guidelines suggest consuming double this amount: about 3 cups (450 g) of fresh legumes or 1 cup (200 g) of dried legumes a week.

NUTS: A SECRET WEAPON FOR WEIGHT LOSS?

As well as being nutritious, nuts help us control our weight.

Don't believe it? I'm not surprised. After all, just 3.5 oz (100 g) of walnuts contains a whopping 689 calories. With all those calories, how can it be possible for nuts to help with weight loss?

Research has found that people can snack on a modest amount of nuts without gaining weight, and that nuts can even help slim us

---

4 Kushi et al., 1999; Curran, 2012
5 Afshin et al., 2014

down due to their **good balance of healthy fats.** Walnuts, almonds, pistachios, hazelnuts, and pine nuts are commonly used in the Mediterranean area, where they easily grow. These nuts have been shown to **protect the cardiovascular system and prevent diabetes,** have **anti-cancer properties** and **anti-aging effects,** and can help **regulate appetite.**

Walnuts in particular are rich in good fats (omega-3 fatty acids), vitamins, phytosterols (which lower LDL cholesterol), fiber, and protein.

Pistachios, compared to the other nuts, are very rich in **phytosterols** (followed by almonds and hazelnuts). Phytosterols are heat resistant, so toasting does not destroy these compounds.

Almonds and **hazelnuts** are rich in **calcium** (240 mg for 3.5 oz or 100 g). For people intolerant to milk and dairy products, these nuts and their products are a great substitute, including the popular almond milk. Almonds are also rich in vitamin E, the undisputed queen among vitamins. Vitamin E has strong antioxidant capacities and can counter the oxidation of LDL cholesterol, a major cause of atherosclerosis. Vitamin E also strengthens the immune system. One serving of almonds (1 oz or 28 g, about 25-30 almonds) provides half the daily requirement of vitamin E.

Pine nuts contain the highest amount of protein of any other nut. Pine nuts also contain a **potent appetite suppressant called pinolenic acid.** Pinolenic acid works by stimulating two hunger-suppressing hormones—**cholecystokinin (CCK) and glucagon-like peptide 1** (GLP-1). CCK is released from the intestine and can actively suppress appetite, promoting a feeling of fullness which reduces further food intake. GLP-1 has a similar effect by slowing down the absorption of food in the intestine. Pine nuts, like all other nuts, are **high fiber foods.** Fiber helps reduce the absorption of sugar, among many other beneficial actions. People who eat high volumes of fiber-rich foods are able to lose weight and maintain a healthy weight easier.

TABLE OF NUTRIENTS: NUTS

	Walnuts (3.5oz–100g)	Pistachios (3.5oz–100g)	Almonds (3.5oz–100g)	Hazelnuts (3.5oz–100g)	Pine nuts (3.5oz–100g)
Energy (calories)	**689**	608	603	655	595
Carbohydrate (g)	5.1	**8.1**	4.6	6.1	4
Protein (g)	14.3	18.3	22	13.8	**31.9**
Fat (g)	**68.1**	56.1	55	64.1	50.3
Fiber (g)	6.2	10.6	**12.7**	8.1	4.5
Vitamin E (mg)	3	4	**26**	15	9.33
Iron (mg)	2.1	**7.3**	3	3.3	2
Calcium (mg)	83	131	**240**	150	40

Nuts are a great and easy snack that gives a sense of satiety and provides many nutrients. **The regular daily serving is ½ -1 oz (14–28 g), about 15–30 nuts (depending on the size).** The table below gives the nutrient content and calorie counts for the most common types of nuts.

SEEDS: THE NATURAL SUPPLEMENT

Seeds are an essential addition to any healthy diet. Smaller and denser than nuts, seeds are filled with **healthy fats (omega-3 fatty acids)**, **protein**, **minerals**, **vitamins**, **fiber**, and **phytonutrients**. Numerous studies have shown that different types of seeds and nuts can actually prevent weight gain, the development of heart disease, and the accumulation of LDL cholesterol. Seeds are the embodiment of a universal life force: each seed, a little powerhouse of massive potential, was destined to grow into an impressive, abundant plant. They are simply bursting with that potential, and they should be part of everybody's daily menu.

If you are going to add seeds to your diet, I would recommend that you eat only organic seeds. I personally love to eat raw seeds; I eat them on a daily basis and they give me a lot of natural energy. They are great if you want a quick, healthy snack that is still low in calories. Obviously, there are many types of seeds, but the seeds listed below are my personal favorites, and the ones which are most common in the Italian diet.

Flax seeds trace their roots back to ancient times, and may have been the world's first cultivated superfood. Flax seed help **improve digestion, lower cholesterol, reduce sugar cravings, balance hormones, fight cancer, and promote weight loss**. Flax seeds, also referred to as linseeds, are small brown, tan, or golden-colored seeds, and are the richest sources of an important plant-based omega-3 FA called alpha-linolenic acid (ALA). One of the most extraordinary benefits of flax seeds is their high levels of **mucilage gum content**. Mucilage is a gel-forming fiber that is water soluble and has incredible benefits for the intestinal tract. It can keep food in the stomach from emptying too quickly into the small intestine, which increases nutrient absorption. Flax seeds are also extremely high in both soluble and insoluble fiber, which can support colon detoxification, fat loss, and reduced sugar cravings.

Sesame seeds are very rich in minerals, **calcium** (100 mg per tablespoon) in particular, and important cholesterol-fighting fibers known as **lignans**. Studies show that these seeds can lower blood pressure as well as protect the liver from damage.

Sunflower seeds are rich in **vitamin E,** an important antioxidant. Balanced levels of vitamin E have been linked to a reduced risk of early death from cardiovascular disease. **Folate**, also found in sunflower seeds, has been shown to promote cardiovascular health from birth to old age and is very important for pregnant women.

Some scientific studies have shown that the components of **pumpkin seeds** may prevent the triggering of **cancerous behavior in male prostate cells**. Pumpkin seeds are high in **carotenoids**, which enhance immune activity and have disease fighting capacities.

Salba-chia seeds, more commonly known as **chia seeds**, are originally from Mexico, but have seen recent popularity in the Italian diet because of their health benefits. These omega-3 FA-rich seeds **help reduce the risk of heart disease and may aid in weight loss and treatment of type 2 diabetes** when consumed in sufficient quantities (about 3 tablespoons, or 180 calories, a day).[6]

SUPPLEMENTS: A POOR ALTERNATIVE TO REAL FOOD

It may seem more practical to take a supplement such as a multivitamin to cover your nutritional needs, but this does not mean that it is the healthier option. It is generally **best to get our vitamins and**

---

6 Vuksan et al., 2017

minerals naturally from the foods we eat (or, in the case of vitamin D, controlled sun exposure).

Recent research on **calcium,** for example, suggests that it is **safest to get calcium from foods** that are naturally rich in calcium, like milk, dairy products, green leafy vegetables, nuts, seeds, and legumes. Elderly women who get high amounts of calcium from supplements have a higher risk of developing kidney stones, stroke, and even death.

There are two **exceptions** to this rule: vitamin B12 and folate. **Vitamin B12** is found exclusively in animal products, so vegans have trouble maintaining their body's stores. Also, between 10–30 percent of elderly people don't properly digest and absorb natural vitamin B12, so it is recommended that these population groups get vitamin B12 from supplements. **Folate,** taken in the form of supplements and fortified foods, is absorbed about 70 percent better than folate found naturally in foods. Consequently, women are advised to get folate from supplements during pregnancy and before conception. Also, keep in mind that for **iron** taken from plant foods or supplements, only around half is absorbed, although eating your spinach with a source of vitamin C, like lemon juice, will slightly boost iron absorption.

Regarding natural versus synthetic forms of vitamins and minerals in dietary supplements, most of the time **natural is better**. Vitamins and bioactive compounds taken in pill form are certainly much less efficient than when they are introduced with foods. The reason for this is that few health benefits can be attributed to a single bioactive compound; rather, it is the **synergy** between different molecules present in plant foods that provide the real benefits. In addition, consuming micronutrients in supplemental form is a missed opportunity for consuming fiber, which has many magnificent health benefits.

Keep in mind that in the case of deficiencies, supplements can help prevent conditions; however, many are known to be harmful in high doses. It is almost impossible to measure your vitamin and mineral intake from foods, so by adding a multivitamin on top of your regular diet may put you at risk of conditions caused by excessive consumption. Before taking any supplement, ask your medical practitioner.

The Mamma Mia Diet is rich in fruits and vegetables, so it can easily provide the daily requirements for vitamins and other micronutrients with extremely low risk of excessive consumption. Unfortunately, people don't always follow a balanced and nutritious diet, and instead take supplements to compensate for a lack of nutrients, not knowing that **good food is the best and cheapest medicine**!

DO's and DON'Ts

If you're having trouble getting the right daily dose of fruits and vegetables, I've tried to simplify things with the following DO's and DON'Ts/LIMITs:

DO's

1. **DO** eat plenty of fresh, seasonal (possibly local) fruits and vegetables every day. Add color, texture, appeal, and health to your plate.
2. **DO** snack on fresh fruits or nuts.
3. **DO** start each meal with a fresh salad dressed with olive oil and lemon juice.
4. **DO** encourage your kids to eat fruits and vegetables by offering it to them each meal and at snack time.
5. **DO** add seeds to your dishes.

DON'Ts/LIMITS

1. **LIMIT** fruit after a large meal. Learn to listen to your body; if fruit sits in the stomach alongside other foods for long enough, fermentation happens, causing bloating and discomfort. If this is you, consume it before the meal or as a snack.
2. **LIMIT** potato consumption, as they are starchy vegetables. Do not combine a meal rich in potatoes with pasta, rice, or bread.
3. **LIMIT** fried vegetables; they are rich in calories.
4. **LIMIT** canned and frozen fruits and vegetables.

SUMMARY

Why eat fruits and vegetables?

Fruit and vegetables are extremely nutritious, containing vitamins, minerals, antioxidants, fiber, and water, which each have different functions contributing to normal body functioning. They are also low in calories, protect from many diseases, and help control weight.

What and how much?

Eating the rainbow (consuming a variety of colors) and eating according to each season is an easy-to-follow guide to eating the proper amount and variety of fruits and vegetables. The daily intake of **fruit** should be two servings, about **4–5 oz (110–140 g) each**: a medium-sized piece of fruit (an apple, a pear, or an orange) or two small fruits (such as plums or apricots).

The daily intake of **vegetables** should be at least three portions. If you consume them **raw**, the serving size should be **2–2.5 oz (60–70 g),** but if we cook them, the **weight before cooking should be 9 oz (about 250 g)**.

When during the day should I eat fruits and vegetables?

Each meal should contain some fruit and plenty of vegetables. It is always good to start our day with a breakfast rich in fruit. Fruit is an excellent snack, too, even better than after a meal.

CHAPTER 5

Fat and the Mamma Mia! Diet

I S FAT BAD OR good? Does fat make us fat?

These are all common questions these days. There is still a lot of confusion about fat, made worse by the misinformation preventing us from taking advantage of the latest studies, which have demonstrated how helpful fat is for losing weight and for general good health. Over the last four decades, fat has been demonized, causing many of us to choose low-fat processed foods where the fat is replaced with salt, sugar, or low-fiber refined grains, rather than increasing our healthy fat intake and learning more about it.

Here, then, is the bottom line: the RIGHT fat in the RIGHT amounts can help us become lean, healthy, and energetic. Fat takes longer to digest than carbohydrates, keeping us fuller longer. This can prevent us from needless eating, which ultimately leads to weight gain. It is sugar (simple sugar), not fat, that steals our health and sabotages our waistline. A high-fat diet with the same caloric content as a high-sugar diet is metabolized differently, and therefore has different physiological effects, which is why high-sugar diets are more strongly associated with cardiovascular disease and diabetes.[1]

---

1 Mozaffarian, 2016

WHAT IS FAT?

The words "lipids" and "fat" are frequently confused, but refer to the same thing: any compound that is not soluble in water but which is soluble in other organic solvents. Think a mix of oil and water—all fats will dissolve in the oil portion, but not in the water. Commonly speaking, we use the term "lipid" to refer to many different molecules such as triglycerides (TG), fatty acids (FAs), cholesterol, and several fat-soluble vitamins (vitamin A, D, E, K), whereas "fat" is more commonly used to describe dietary fat, one of the three macronutrients (carbohydrates, fat, and protein) which mostly encompasses fatty acids in the form of triglycerides. The latest nutritional guidelines suggest that in a balanced diet, dietary fat should account for 30 percent of total energy intake.

During its metabolism, fat provides about 9 calories/gram.

Saturated and Unsaturated Fatty Acids

Saturated fats and unsaturated fats are found in a variety of foods and fall into one of four categories:

Saturated fatty acids have no double bonds between the carbons in their chains, and are most commonly present in animal products (meat, milk, cheese, butter) and some oils from tropical plants, such as palm oil and coconut oil.

Monounsaturated fatty acids (MUFAs) contain one double bond between two carbon atoms and are present most commonly in vegetable oil (such as olive and canola oil).

Polyunsaturated fatty acids (PUFAs) contain two or more double bonds between carbon atoms and are found in fish, nuts, and seeds. The PUFAs **linoleic acid** (LA) and **alpha-linolenic acid** (ALA) are the only essential dietary fatty acids; while they are necessary for proper growth and development, our bodies cannot make them naturally. Our cells are capable of using these two fatty acids to synthesize other fatty acids such as arachidonic acid (AA), eicosapentaenoic acid

(EPA), and docosahexaenoic acid (DHA). For this reason, these three fatty acids are called **essential fatty acids,** because while our bodies need them, we can make them if and only if we are consuming LA and ALA. Although society tends to lump these fatty acids together by simply referring to them as omega-6 or omega-3, all of these fatty acids have different roles in our body. Therefore, it is very important that we include all of them in our diet, which can be done by eating a well-balanced diet, full of a variety of food.

Trans **fatty acids** can be natural or artificial, though they are mostly artificially created through a process known as **hydrogenation** (which involves heating and a chemical structure change, making the fatty acid more saturated). Artificial *trans* fatty acids are found in any food that has hydrogenated oil as an ingredient, such as commercially baked products and packaged foods such as cookies, pie crust, baked food, and frostings. They are also found in fast foods, specifically fried foods and deep-fried food, and are considered the most unhealthy fats (even worse than saturated fats). Natural *trans* fatty acids can be found in small amounts in milk, beef, and cheese, but these should not be anything to worry about.

WHY DO WE NEED FAT?

Fats are frequently disparaged as the cause of several health problems, including obesity and cardiovascular disease, giving the impression that fat should be avoided.

As stated previously, fats are important in our diet for a number of reasons:

1 **Energy.** Our bodies need energy for survival, and dietary fat can be used after consumption as a source of energy. It can also be stored in the adipose tissue for future use.

2 **Proper functioning of nerves and brain.** Fats are part of **myelin,** a fatty substance that wraps around our nerve cells, allowing them to send electrical messages.

3 **Maintaining proper cell membranes.** The maintenance of our cell's membrane allows for the efficient exchange of nutrients and removal of waste.

4 **Transporting fat-soluble vitamins A, D, E, and K through the bloodstream.** Without fat, these vitamins cannot be absorbed. A low-fat diet compromises fat-soluble vitamin absorption; in fact, you can increase your fat-soluble vitamin absorption by consuming fat with every meal.

5 **Forming steroid hormones.** Hormones are compounds that help regulate the necessary bodily processes. Fats, specifically cholesterol, help form these compounds.

6 **Providing flavor to food.** Good fats give our foods flavor and texture that, without it, would leave us with a bland and dry diet.

7 **Serve as precursors to other necessary regulatory compounds.** PUFAs are utilized by the body to make compounds called **oxylipins**, which are involved in inflammatory and developmental pathways, along with other necessary body functions.

BUTTER AND CHEESE

Butter is delicious! It is one of those foods that can turn bland meals into masterpieces. In desserts, it adds a special flavor that no vegetable oil can reproduce. Despite having been demonized in the past, **good butter** (especially from grass-fed cows) is actually **healthy,** containing various beneficial compounds such as **vitamins A, E, and K2**; **conjugated linoleic acid (CLA),** which has powerful effects on metabolism (and is actually sold commercially as a weight loss supplement); and **3–4% butyric acid**, which is anti-in-flammatory and has powerful protective effects on the digestive system.[2]

Butter in moderation is fine, but like with any food, it may cause health problems if you eat way too much (for example, by adding a few tablespoons to your morning toast every day or your bread during meals). When I bake, I will usually reduce the amount of butter instead of replacing it with margarine, for example, because margarine is highly processed and contains *trans* fatty acids.

When it comes to **cheese**, on the other hand, you'll likely have either heard it's very good for you, or that it can make you fat and is something to avoid completely. Neither extreme provides a fair picture of cheese. The truth is actually somewhere in the middle, like every-thing in life. **Cheese is a great source of calcium and protein**. It also contains some **vitamins (such as vitamins A and B12) and minerals (such as zinc and phosphorus)**. A recent study in the

2 Säemann MD et al., 2000

European Journal of Clinical Nutrition[3] showed that both sheep's milk and goat's milk lower bad cholesterol (LDL), are anti-inflammatory, and may protect against cardio-vascular disease and colon cancer.

Cheese is a high-fat and high-calorie food. Depending on the variety of cheese you eat, you're getting about 100 calories per ounce, or 28 g (for seasoned cheese), and about 6–9 grams of fat, mostly saturated. It's also loaded with sodium. That said, you shouldn't be afraid to add cheese to your meals, especially if you are using **fresh (not processed) cheeses like ricotta, feta, cottage cheese, and mozzarella (semi-fat cheese)**. Cheese contains also lactose, a sugar that can't be digested by lactose-intolerant people because they lack an enzyme called **lactase**. However, this is not the case with Italian **Parmesan cheese;** 6–8 hours after the cheese is made, the **lactose is transformed into easy-to-digest lactic acid** through the action of enzymes in the cheese.

As a side note, **yogurt** can also be part of a **lactose-free diet.** Yogurt has live cultures that convert lactose to lactic acid. Yogurt appears protective against diabetes and weight gain, which may be due to its probiotic content, and is something to include in your daily menu. In Mediterranean countries, yogurt is a very popular ingredient, and makes for a tasty dessert with fruit (for more info, refer to Part III: Desserts) or a perfect food for breakfast and snacks. It can also be consumed as a drink or turned into a delicious cheese.

---

3 Pes GM et al., 2015

SATURATED FAT VS UNSATURATED FAT: WHICH SHOULD WE CHOOSE?

Recent studies suggest that unsaturated fats alone may not be as heart healthy as we once thought, and that consuming saturated fats may not be as dangerous as once thought.

There has already been ample evidence provided by scientific research that a healthy diet should introduce **a correct proportion of saturated and unsaturated fats**. The Italian guidelines suggest getting no more than 10 percent of your daily calories from saturated fat. In fact, a recent epidemiological study indicated that higher dietary intakes of saturated fats is associated with an increased risk of coronary heart disease. The authors of the study found that the risk of coronary heart disease is significantly lower when replacing saturated fats with unsaturated fats and choosing whole grain carbohydrates or plant proteins.[4] However, it is hard to draw any sound conclusions from epidemiological studies, since nothing is being controlled for; correlation is not causation. What we can conclude is that a dietary shift towards "whole," less processed foods can lead to better health.

Regardless, it is best to never simply eliminate anything from your diet. My recommendation to you is to eat everything in moderation, including saturated and unsaturated fats, because that will ensure that you are getting a variety of nutrients.

TYPES OF UNSATURATED FATS

Not all unsaturated fats are created equal. **Soybean oil, sunflower oil, corn oil, and safflower oil,** for example, are **processed oils** created by the food industry. In the U.S., they will typically use genetically modified crops and high heat during production which can produce benzopyrenes, which have been shown to be carcinogenic.

---

4 Zong G. et al, 2016

Lower quality oils may also be extracted using chemical methods, such as solvents, which negatively affects taste and can be toxic if consumed in high quantities. These oils are **less healthy,** and contain different proportions of fatty acids, which all have different physiological effects.

Canola Oil

So, which unsaturated fatty acid *should* you introduce in a healthy diet? Certainly **oleic acid (a monounsaturated fat) is an excellent choice,** and this which can be found in the highest concentrations in **canola oil** and especially **olive oil.**

Canola oil was first created by Canadian scientists, and was obtained from rapeseed oil normally used for industrial purposes, which people couldn't eat due to some unfavorable substances such as erucic acid, a fatty acid that has shown to cause heart damage in some rat studies, and glucosinolates, bitter compounds that made the oil taste bad.

The scientists used selective breeding techniques to "create" seeds that contained less of these compounds and more oleic acid, as well as PUFAs. Today, about 90% of the world's canola crop is genetically modified. Typical fatty acid composition of canola oil is **6% saturated fat, 62% monounsaturated fat, and 29% polyunsaturated fat.**[5] Currently, there is no evidence of toxic compounds present in canola oil; however, in my opinion, it is clearly better to use other types of oils rich in saturated fat (like coconut oil).

Olive Oil

That said, **olive oil** is certainly *the choice* when it comes to healthy oil. For many food lovers, nothing is more appreciated than the

5 Richardson et al. 2017

exquisite taste of top-quality extra virgin olive oil. Organically produced, extra virgin olive oil is almost indescribable in its rich taste and aroma.

Olive oil has been an integral part of the Mediterranean culture for centuries, not only because of its delicious flavor but also due to its health benefits. In the past, olive oil was actually used as a medicine in addition to being used for culinary purposes. Generally, Italian oil producers strive for full-bodied, green-colored olive oil, often with small, visible sediments and a slightly herbal aroma. This differs from olive oil produced in the United States, which instead aims to be more neutral and clear in color. Because olive oil contains unsaturated fatty acids, it should be stored away from sunlight in a cool place.

Extra Virgin Olive Oil

Extra virgin olive oil is the **highest grade** of olive oil. It is produced using only pressure and without refinement, meaning **no heat-cold pressed**! Extra virgin olive oil also has a higher volume of phenolic antioxidants compared to its lower-quality counterparts, which help protect the oil from oxidation. When introduced into the body, antioxidants can help prevent LDL cholesterol from oxidation, promoting a healthier balance of cholesterol, and fight systemic inflammation, which is responsible for several preventable diseases including cardiovascular disease and diseases associated with the aging process. Recently, Dr. Panico from the Temple University of Philadelphia has shown (in animal models) that chronic administration of a diet enriched with extra virgin olive oil induces an improvement of working memory and spatial learning. In particular, olive oil from the Apulia region in Italy seems to have a protective action against the onset of Alzheimer's disease. Extra virgin olive oil contains **16% saturated fat (mainly palmitic acid, 14%); 73% monounsaturated**

fat (mainly oleic acid, 71%) and 10% polyunsaturated fat (mainly linoleic acid, 9%).[6]

The best ways to incorporate olive oil into your diet include:

- Drizzle it on cooked vegetables and soups
- Mix with chopped garlic, lemon juice, and sea salt for your salad dressing
- Instead of buttering your bread, dip it into extra virgin olive oil. It was one of my favorite afternoon snacks when I was a kid!
- Sauté and stir-fry vegetables in olive oil; this gives it a special taste and is an excellent choice for pan-frying.

Palm Oil

There has been so much talk lately about palm oil and whether it's good or bad for you. **Palm oil** derives from the fleshy fruit of oil palms; used for cooking, it is also added to many ready-to-eat foods. The fatty acid composition of **palm oil is: unsaturated (45–55%); monounsaturated (38–45%); and polyunsaturated (9–12%).**

In the past few years, palm oil has come under fire for containing high percentages of saturated fatty acids, supposedly **raising blood cholesterol and increasing the risk of cardiovascular disease** as a result.[7]

However, international guidelines (in agreement with recent studies) indicate that the consumption of palm oil as a source of dietary saturated fat does *not* add any additional risks for cardiovascular disease when consumed in moderation as part of a

6 Richardson et al., 2017
7 Clarke et al., 1997; Jensen et al., 1999

well-balanced diet. Remember that the recommended intake of saturated fat is less than 10% of total daily calories.[8]

According to Harvard nutrition experts, "Palm oil is better than *trans* FAs, but vegetable oils such as olive oil and canola oil should still be the first choices."

For the Mamma Mia Diet, there's no question—extra virgin cold pressed olive oil is certainly the best choice!

Coconut Oil

Recently, there has been a dietary trend recommending the use of **coconut oil** in place of traditional oils for cooking processes. This may sound confusing, because coconut oil, like butter, is mostly saturated fat, something we are told to decrease in our diets.

These claims started due to the unique fatty acid content of coconut oil. Coconut oil, unlike most other oils, contains mostly medium chain fatty acids (MCFAs), which consist of 8–10 carbons, as opposed to long chain fatty acids, which consist of more than ten carbons. The body metabolizes MCFAs differently because we lack an enzyme that can "place" them onto chylomicrons, which are the lipid transport proteins that transport just-eaten fatty acids from our small intestine to the rest of the body. Instead, these MCFAs are transported directly to the liver, where they are incorporated into VLDL, or used immediately by the liver.

Recent studies have shown that replacing other dietary oils with coconut oil, despite its high saturated fat content, can **increase HDL cholesterol (the "good" cholesterol) and decrease waist circumference**.[9] However, because this is a "new" culinary trend, we are unaware if there are any long-term adverse effects of a diet rich in coconut oil, so **use this oil in moderation.**

8 Mukherjee and Mitra 2009; Marangoni et al., 2017
9 Cardoso et al. 2015

Omega-3s and Omega-6s

We've already mentioned them numerous times, but what exactly are omega-3 and omega-6 fatty acids, and how much of them should we be consuming?

Simply put, omega-3 and omega-6 fatty acids are **polyunsaturated fatty acids (PUFAs)** essential to the human body that serve as precursors to important cell signaling molecules.

There are three main omega-3 FAs: **eicosapentaenoic acid (EPA), docosahexaenoic acid (DHA)**, which comes mainly from fish, and **alpha-linolenic acid (ALA)**, found in vegetable oils (especially soybean and canola), nuts (especially walnuts), seeds, and leafy vegetables.

Much of the current scientific research suggests that omega-3 FAs affect many beneficial actions: **neuroprotection, anti-hypertension, anti-hyperalgesia, anti-arrhythmia,** and **anti-tumorigenesis,** to name a few.[10]

Experimental data also shows that omega-3 FAs exert their protective effects **against ischemic injury (partly through inhibiting oxidative stress) and possess therapeutic potential for a variety of neurological disorders, including ischemic stroke.**[11] Omega-3-derived compounds are also mediators of the inflammatory process and tend to be associated with anti-inflammatory actions.

Omega-6 and omega-3 also both play a crucial role in brain function, and normal growth and development, though the two accomplish this through opposite means. Omega-3s help **reduce** inflammation, while some omega-6s tend to **promote** inflammation. For this reason, guidelines suggest a **correct ratio between omega-6 and omega-3 of 4:1.** The best way to get an adequate amount of both fatty acids is to eat a wide variety of fats.

---

10 KudaO, 2017
11 ShiZ et al., 2016

Unfortunately, the typical American diet tends to contain 14–25 times more omega-6 than omega-3. In fact, over the past century, the consumption of omega-6, specifically in the form of linoleic acid (LA), has significantly increased, most likely due to increased consumption of vegetable oils high in LA, like soybean and corn oil.[12] The Mamma Mia Diet, which is based on the Mediterranean diet, has a better balance between omega-6 and omega-3 FAs. The MMD also does not include much meat (which is high in omega-6,) and emphasizes consuming foods rich in omega-3s, including whole grains, fresh fruits and vegetables, and fish.

WHAT IS THE BEST FAT FOR FRYING?

Dear Mr. Fried Food, why are you so good? Biologically speaking, we are predisposed to enjoy more energy-dense foods—foods high in fat and/or sugar—and fried fat fits in this category. Deep-frying is a cooking method that involves submerging a food in hot fat. The ideal temperature of the oil is around 350–375°F (180–190°C). When the temperature is too low, the fat will seep into the food, making it greasy; when the temperature is too high, it can dry out the food and oxidize the fat.

While fried food tastes good, it is certainly not good for our health. It's fine to splurge and enjoy yourself once in a while, but try to do so at home to minimize some of its unhealthful effects. Choose your cooking fat carefully. Fats with high "smoke points" react less with oxygen and are the best oils for frying. The **smoke point** of an oil is the temperature at which, under specific and defined conditions, it begins to produce a continuous smoke that

12 Blasbalg et al. 2011

becomes clearly visible. You should also pan-fry whenever possible. The more saturated the fats are, the more stable they are when heated. When it comes to pan-frying, however, the temperature is much lower and less oil is used, making it a healthier alternative to deep-fat frying.

Coconut oil is a good choice for pan-frying. Over 90 percent of the fatty acids in coconut oil are saturated, which makes it very resistant to heat. However, food fried in coconut oil will absorb high amount of it, making the resulting dish rich in saturated fat.

Olive oil, as we've said, is **one of the healthiest fat on earth.** It is very high in monounsaturated fatty acids, which have only one double bond. Like saturated fats, monounsaturated fats are highly resistant to heat. Olive oil is a good option for pan-frying, as well; look for a mildly flavored olive oil! Other oils to consider include **avocado oil**, which is similar to olive oil but has a unique taste making it unpopular in a Mediterranean-style diet; and **peanut oil,** which has a neutral taste and a high smoke point, but is relatively high in polyunsaturated fats, which makes it vulnerable to oxidative damage at high temperatures.

There are several fats and oils that I recommend you **not** use. These include **vegetable oils** that are high in linoleic acid, such as **soybean**, **safflower, sunflower, and corn oil**, as this will upset your ratio.

As an aside, **lard** is also a very good frying fat, because the majority of its fatty acids are saturated and monounsaturated, making it very resistant to high heat. It was commonly used in the past in many cuisines, but now it being used less because it has a strong, distinct taste that can cover the food's flavor.

CHOLESTEROL: FRIEND OR FOE?

We hear so much about the dangers of high cholesterol through the media and the risks it poses to our long-term health. But what is cholesterol?

Cholesterol is a lipid molecule present in all cells of the body. It can be found in the foods we eat, but our bodies also make cholesterol because it is an essential compound needed for life. It is an essential component of our cell membranes, it modulates membrane fluidity, and is also the precursor of hormones, vitamin D, and bile (important for digestion).

Our body actually makes all the cholesterol that it needs. Nevertheless, cholesterol is found in many animal foods, so we tend to end up with more than we need. Vegetables contain phytosterols, which have a different chemical structure compared to cholesterol and, for this reason, cannot be used by animal cells.

For years, the public has believed that lowering dietary cholesterol will dramatically decrease our blood cholesterol levels, which is why we've all heard that lowering our dietary cholesterol levels is the thing to do. However, our body actually makes relatively **high** amounts of cholesterol; the amount of cholesterol in the average diet pales in comparison to what our body makes. Additionally, **studies have shown that decreasing dietary cholesterol actually causes the body to produce more cholesterol as a response**. With that understanding, dietary cholesterol is not something that you should concern yourself with.

Regarding the monikers "good" and "bad" cholesterol: there are two types of lipoproteins that carry cholesterol in the bloodstream: low-density lipoproteins (LDL) and high-density lipoproteins (HDL). LDL-cholesterol is usually called "**bad cholesterol**" because it is high in fat and cholesterol, and is not very dense (hence the term "low-density"). LDL is what transports cholesterol from the liver to the rest of the body, and is the lipoprotein most associated with the development of atherosclerosis. **HDL-cholesterol**, usually called

"good cholesterol," is thought to be heart-protective because it transports fats from the body to the liver, meaning it takes cholesterol out of transport. It is important to note that having healthy levels of both types of lipoproteins is important, as we need both for survival. The Mamma Mia Diet, filled as it is with a lot of fruits, vegetables, whole grains, legumes, and fish, along with olive oil, a moderate intake of saturated fat, *trans* fats, and dietary cholesterol (and 1–2 glasses of red wine a day) is a ***cholesterol-lowering,*** **heart-healthy eating plan**.

DO's and DON'Ts

Having trouble getting your daily dose of healthy fat? To make it easier, I've summarized the key points of this chapter into some DO's and DON'Ts/LIMITs:

DO's

1. **DO** eat extra-virgin oil. It is the number one fat choice, but quantity is important, too. The MMD recommends a daily intake of about 4–5 tablespoons (60–75 g) per day for a male adult, and 3–4 tablespoons (45–60 g) for a female adult.
2. **DO** adopt healthy cooking methods (refer to Appendix A: Cooking Techniques).
3. **DO** eat a variety of nuts and seeds.
4. **DO** eat fish rich in omega-3 FAs.
5. **DO** eat cheese, but only in moderation. I recommend you stay away from cheeses where the manufacturers have purposefully added unnecessary salt and chemicals. Look for genuine cheeses (preferably fresh), not imitation cheese products.
6. **DO** read labels and stay away from food with *trans* and hydrogenated fatty acids.

DON'Ts/LIMITS

1. **DON'T** eat the same fat every day.
2. **DON'T** eat fried food, or if you must, only occasionally and homemade.
3. **DON'T** eat fast food, which is rich in bad fat (*trans* fatty acids).

4. **DON'T** eat processed food, especially foods labeled as "light," because generally the fat will have been replaced with sugar.

5. **LIMIT** mayonnaise (replace it with strained yogurt).

6. **LIMIT** whipped cream with your sweets, coffee or hot chocolate. Ideally, make your own whipped cream and add less sugar.

SUMMARY

Why eat fat?
Fat is both an energy source and energy storage. It allows for proper functioning of nerves and the brain, and is a major structural component of cell membranes. It helps transport fat-soluble vitamins A, D, E, and K through the bloodstream, is the precursor for signaling molecules as well as steroid hormones, and it enhances food flavor. In short? Fat does a *lot!*

What and how much fat should I eat?
Fats should be **30% of our daily caloric intake,** of which 80–90% should be **unsaturated** and with a very low amount of ***trans*** fatty acids.

When during the day should I eat fat?
Each meal should include a certain percentage of fat to help cover our daily intake.

CHAPTER 6

Protein and the Mamma Mia! Diet

ROTEIN IS AN IMPORTANT component of every cell in the body. Along with carbs and fat, protein is the third and final "macronutrient" (vitamins and minerals, which are needed in only small amounts, are called "micronutrients"). Although typically when we think about protein, we think of meat, protein is not only found in meat; there are other sources of protein available, including fish, certain vegetables, eggs, and dairy.

PROTEIN: AN OVERVIEW

A Dutch chemist in 1838 coined the term "protein," drawing on the Greek word "*proteios*," which means "the first quality." And in fact, **proteins** are the **fundamental basis of life** on this planet. Comprised of long chains made up of twenty amino acids that can be arranged in millions of different ways to create millions of different proteins, each protein is unique, with its own specific function.

The reason why protein is one of the most important nutrients in the human diet is because our body does not synthesize nine of these amino acids. These amino acids are called "**essential amino acids**," because it is essential that we obtain them from our diet.

All dietary protein contains some of these twenty amino acids, but they are found in different proportions. Foods that contain the nine essential amino acids, in the correct proportions that correspond to human body needs, are called "**complete proteins**" and generally come from animal sources. Foods that are lacking in one or more of the essential amino acids relative to our needs are called "**incomplete proteins**."

As to the role it plays in our lives, think of protein as **the building blocks of our body**. When you build a house, you need good, solid materials to build with; otherwise, the house will not be very solid. Protein is absolutely essential for the growth and repair of our tissues, as well as building hormones (like insulin), enzymes (like digestive enzymes), and antibodies. Whatever we are (carnivores, pescatarians, vegetarians, or vegans) protein should always be present in our daily diet.

During its metabolism, protein provides 4 calories per gram.

Animal vs Vegetable Protein

Protein is essential to our survival and the most plentiful and accessible sources of complete proteins are found in animal sources. Yet many people, for reasons of health or conscience, do not eat animal products, or eat them only rarely.

Our intestine does not care whether the protein we consume is from animal or vegetable sources; however, as mentioned above, the important point is how many and which essential amino acids are introduced. If we do not consume the essential amino acids, we will not synthesize enough protein for our bodies to function correctly.

Relative to animal products (meat, dairy, and eggs), vegetables tend to have relatively lower concentrations of proteins and usually have some, but not all of the essential amino acids. An exception to this rule is soybeans and, to a lesser extent, legumes (for more information, see the section on page 74, "The Soybean Controversy).

Whole grains also contain respectable levels of protein but are similarly incomplete.

To overcome this problem, eating foods from different plants in **combination** with other protein sources can provide the right amount of protein we need. To elaborate: a food may be lacking in one essential amino acid, but when consumed with another food that **is** high in that amino acid, the amino acid profiles of the food "complement" each other and create a complete protein. A good example of this is the combination of legumes and cereals. The nutritional deficiencies in each are well compensated for; you'll find this type of combination is common in many Italian peasant dishes because meat was not always available.

The idea of complementary foods was first discovered by accident by primitive farmers. This is one of socio-evolutionary reasons explaining why civilization started from three areas of the world: Latin America (where beans and corn were grown), central Asia (soybean and rice) and the Mediterranean area (cereals and *fava* beans, as well as chickpeas and lentils).

My personal choice is to mix animal and vegetable protein, making deliberate decisions based on the type and the source, preferring local products. While I am not vegetarian, I do have some meat free days (usually Monday and Friday); it is my hope that more people make an effort to choose to eat plant-based protein, which will lead to a decline in the production of meat and the development of a more sustainable feeding model.

THE SOYBEAN CONTROVERSY

Yes, there are so many different opinions on the topic of soybeans that we can easily get confused—especially in Italy, where soybean is a pretty new ingredient to our cuisine, arriving by way of China only in the nineteenth century.

Soybean is a type of legume, and is an important component of the Asian diet. Many products can be obtained using soybeans, including soymilk, oil, tofu, and tempeh. Soybean is an example of a plant-based complete protein. The major proteins are glycinin and conglycinin, which may trigger allergic reactions in some people. The fat content is mainly polyunsaturated (linoleic acid) and monounsaturated FAs, with small amounts of saturated FAs. The carbs present in soybeans have a very low GI, making soybeans particularly suitable for diabetics. Soybeans are also fairly high in fiber and are a good source of vitamins (B1, K, and folate) and minerals. Another great component of soybeans is its bioactive plant compound content: isoflavones, saponins, and biopeptides.

Several studies have shown that consumption of soybeans has a beneficial impact on the risk factors for cardiovascular disease and levels of LDL and HDL cholesterol.[1] Other studies indicate that consumption of soybean foods is associated with a reduction in prostate cancer risk in men and postmenopausal osteoporosis in woman.[2]

---

1 Hecker, 2001
2 Yan and Spitznagel, 2009; Messina, 2014.

However, recent studies done in the last few years have questioned the health benefits of soybeans. First, the *type* of soy product is important. Over 90 percent of soybeans produced in the U.S. are genetically modified, and the crops are sprayed with pesticides. Second, the *quantity* of soybean foods consumed is also essential to achieve the health effects.[3] Finally, in some people, soy products elicit adverse effects, such as allergies and the suppression of thyroid function. Isoflavones, which soybeans contain, also function as **goitrogens**, which are substances that interfere with thyroid function. They inhibit the function of the enzyme thyroid peroxidase, which is essential for production of thyroid hormones, leading to hypothyroidism and obesity. Isoflavones can also function as phytoestrogens that can activate estrogen receptors in the human body. Due to the estrogenic activity, isoflavones are often used as a natural alternative to estrogenic drugs to relieve symptoms of menopause.

Although soybean is certainly an important substitute for meat as protein source, the existing data is not sufficient to support most of the suggested health benefits of consuming soybean protein or isoflavones.

---

3 Chao, 2008

Protein and Dieting

Some well-known diets advocate high protein consumption for fast weight loss or building muscle. But is this really possible?

The answer is yes, this is possible in the short term, but with serious side effects in the long term. Protein is important, but some diets overestimate the power of protein and advocate high protein consumption for fast weight loss, building muscles, and general well-being. Bodybuilders, for example, eat large quantities of meat and consume synthetic protein with drinks and shakes to build up bigger and stronger muscles.

Further complicating things, most of the diets based on high protein content practically exclude carbohydrates (such as the Atkins diet and the Paleo diet).

And certainly, if we follow these diets we can lose weight in a short period of time (with a lot of gratification along the way), but if we continue this regime for a long period, it **can be harmful**. Without carbs, our body has to get energy from elsewhere—for example, breaking down fats and proteins, which can lead to a physiological state called **ketosis**. If too many stored fats are broken down for energy, ketones build up within the body. As ketone levels rise, acidity of the blood rises, leading to **ketoacidosis**, a serious condition that can cause brain damage, kidney failure, and seizures. Additionally, most of the weight that is lost during the initial stages of a low-carb diet is actually due to water loss, not fat loss, meaning that while your scale might say you are losing weight, you have really just lost water.

Animal Protein

The quality of the protein in any animal is the same because they are all a complete protein. The old expression "Fewer legs is better protein" doesn't hold water. The major difference in comparing the quality of animal meat is the fat content.

Fish is a great source of good protein and omega-3 FAs (1 serving = 5–6 oz or 140–170 g). For example, 4 oz of salmon (110 g) **provides 30 g of protein** and 16 g of fat, where **only 3 g are saturated.** Since Italy is a country with thousands of miles of coastline, it is understandable that fish is a big part of our diet. Little fishes like sardines, anchovies, and mackerels (called *"pesce azzurro"* in Italian) are cheap and abundant in Mediterranean waters and are a good source of omega-3 FAs. Bigger fish like tuna, salmon, cod fish, and sea bass are also featured regularly, as well as shellfish and octopus. I recommend eating fish and seafood grilled, baked, steamed, or pan-fried with olive oil. (In Part III: Recipes and Seasonal Menus, you can find many of my favorite fish dishes!)

Chicken is a **wonderful source of protein (1 serving is equal to 4–5 oz or 110–140 g).** Chicken consists of high-quality protein: 4 oz (or 110 g) contains **34 g of protein,** with eight essential amino acids and a relatively **low amount of fat.** Chicken is also versatile in the kitchen—hot or cold, chicken is an easy ingredient for many ready-in-a-minute meals. Chicken is also a common ingredient in the Italian diet; it easily blends seasonings and spices (in Part III: Recipes and Seasonal Menus you can find many chicken dishes). Plus, when your recipe calls for a type of meat that is too costly or not available, chicken is always a reliable substitute. But never mix chicken with pasta; this combination is *not* classical Italian!

Red meat, which has a darker color than white meat due to its higher levels of oxygen-binding proteins, includes beef, lamb, and pork. **Red and processed meat** have a bad reputation because high consumption of these types of meat has **been associated with colorectal cancer risk.**[4] However, a lean beef steak contains high biological value protein; **4 oz (110 g) contains 32 g of protein.** It also contains **a lot of fat (about 30 g), 10 g of which is saturated.** This is another reason to reduce consumption, but red meat remains an

4 Bernstein et al., 2015

important source of micronutrients including **B vitamins**, **iron** and **zinc.** If you like red meat, **choose lean cuts and smaller portions (about 3.5–4 oz or 100–110 g)** and try to eat it rarely, preferring fish and chicken as source of animal protein.

Processed meat includes bacon, sausages, hot dogs, salami, corned beef, beef jerky, and ham, as well as canned meat and meat-based sauces. It is a type of meat (mainly comprising of pork and beef) that has been modified by methods such as smoking, curing, or adding salt or preservatives. **Potentially carcinogenic chemicals** can form during meat processing,[5] including **N-nitroso compounds and polycyclic aromatic hydrocarbons**. Cooking meat at high temperatures, especially on a barbecue, can also produce these dangerous chemicals (for more information, refer to Appendix A: "Cooking Techniques"). The **consumption of processed meat should be reduced to small amounts weekly** (one serving should not be more than 1.8 oz or 50 g) according to the evaluation of the International Agency for Research on Cancer (IARC) in October 2015. That said, cold cuts like *"salame," "prosciutto crudo,"* and *"pancetta" are* staples of Italian cuisine, and definitely something to try when you are in Italy. The type and preparation varies from region to region, ranging from a milder taste in the north to a spicier one in the south. Two or three slices of good *"salame"* or *"prosciutto crudo"* once in a while with a glass of red wine will not kill you. But it should be a treat—not a habit!

5　Bernstein et al., 2015

TABLE OF ANIMAL PROTEIN

Meat Protein Source (4 oz or 110 g)	Amount of Protein
Fish (such as salmon)	30 g
Chicken	34 g
Lean beef	32 g
Lean pork	29 g

VEGETARIANISM AND VEGANISM

Is it true that if we want to become centenarians we should become vegetarians? Or even vegans?

In the scientific community, the controversy regarding omnivorous, vegetarian, and vegan diets and their effects on aging are still ongoing.

Two important studies confirmed and expanded on the relationship between the risk of cardiovascular disease, the intake of animal foods, and the potentially protective role of fruit and vegetable consumption.[6] Observational studies suggest that a plant-based diet high in fiber-rich foods, such as vegetables, fruits, cereals, whole grains, and legumes, is inversely related to overweight BMIs; semi-vegetarian, lacto-vegetarian, and vegan women have a lower risk of becoming overweight and obese than do omnivorous women.[7]

Studies have also shown that most centenarians have a genetic variation that allows for two key characteristics that may be

6 Stamler, 1979; Yusuf et al., 2004
7 Newby et al., 2005

contributing to their long life. The first is that all centenarians love bitter foods (like arugula, kale, and most vegetables in general); and the second is that they have a better ability to absorb the nutrients within those foods. This, however, is observational data and warrants further investigation of the subject.[8]

The American Dietetic Association has established that a vegetarian diet, one that does not exclude dairy and eggs, is sustainable and safe for all age groups and in all physiological conditions.[9]

DAIRY AS A SOURCE OF PROTEIN

Is dairy a good source of protein? Why do so many diets condemn dairy, especially milk?

Milk is a very complex food because it contains both macronutrients (protein, fat and sugar) and micronutrients (calcium, along with other vitamins and minerals). It also contains **growth factors** that are potentially capable of regulating the body's physiology, as well as **micro-RNA** molecules. This topic is part of several recent studies, whose physiological role is not yet fully clarified[10]. In particular, there are some bioactive peptides with **anti-hypertensive, anti-thrombotic, stimulant properties**[11]. In regards to fat composition, whole milk contains **cholesterol** and **saturated FAs**, whereas in low-fat milk, the percentage of fat is lower. Sugar (lactose) and **vitamins (especially vitamins D and A)** are present, as well. Finally, milk contains a great amount of **calcium (about 120 mg per 100 ml)**. The "calcium reservoirs" found in bone are primarily built in the first decade of life, which is what makes milk so important for children and elderly people, as well.

---

8 Campa et al., 2012
9 Craig et al., 2009
10 Melnik et al., 2016
11 Bouglé and Bouhallab , 2017

Regarding calcium intake, most guidelines indicate **800/1100 mg** of calcium daily[12], drawn from different types of food such as dried fruits, vegetables, and a serving of milk per day. Recent scientific studies have demonstrated that increased calcium intake in the form of supplements has small, inconsistent benefits on fracture prevention and is not risk-free. Indeed, the intake of 1000 mg from supplements has been associated with an increased risk of heart attack, stroke, kidney stones, and gastrointestinal symptoms.[13]

In recent years, milk has become increasingly discussed by the media, with people asserting that our species continued daily consumption of milk is unique to humans, and therefore unnatural. To that, I would say that only goes to show that our evolution is inimitable; we are also the only animals to peel fruits and to cook them!

Based on a systematic review of the epidemiological literature, the World Cancer Research Fund and the American Institute for Cancer Research Report concluded that there was a **probable** association between milk intake and **lower risk of colorectal cancer**, a **probable** association between **diets high in calcium and increased risk of prostate cancer**, and **limited evidence** of an association between milk intake and **lower risk of bladder cancer**. For other cancers, evidence was mixed or lacking.

Recently, the EPIC-Oxford Study demonstrated that:

1. **Dairy products** have a possible **protective role in colorectal cancer risk**.

2. **High yogurt intake** is significantly associated with **decreased colorectal cancer risk**, suggesting that yogurt should be part of any diet meant to prevent the disease. Moreover, the large multicenter study suggest that there is no association between dietary fat and prostate cancer risk.[14]

---

12 Italian LARN, 2014
13 Tai et al., 2015
14 Crowe et al., 2008; Pala et al., 2011; Murphy et al., 2013

It should also be noted that in the U.S., many people purchase low-fat or non-fat milk to avoid excessive fat consumption or because they are watching their calorie intake. Despite this, it would be more beneficial for people to choose whole milk, because it allows for increased absorption of the various fat-soluble vitamins found in milk like vitamins A and D. Vitamin D plays a vital role in calcium absorption, meaning if you want to maximize your calcium absorption and decrease your risk of developing osteoporosis, simply drink whole milk! (It also tastes much better!)

In conclusion, **milk and dairy are high quality foods, rich in macro- and micro-nutrients**. The American guidelines **suggest 1–2 servings /day of milk and/or yogurt, which are similar to the Italian Guidelines (LARN) that suggest the consumption of 2–3 servings of milk or yogurt per day (an Italian serving size is half that of a U.S. serving)**.

EGGS: HEALTHY OR NOT?

It seems like every week brings with it a new controversy about eating **eggs**.

Eggs are among the few foods that you may classify as **"superfoods."** Indeed, eggs are an excellent source of **protein (6 g/egg)** because they contain **all the essential amino acids** in the right ratios. One egg also has varying amounts of **13 essential vitamins**; in particular vitamins A, D, and B12, and minerals such as **selenium, iron, calcium, and choline**. All of this for **only 70 calories**! Isn't it amazing?

Eggs also contain **carotenoids** (lutein and zeaxanthin), powerful antioxidants that protect against age-related macular degeneration and cataracts.[15] All these nutrients indicate that **eggs are an excellent food choice**. The **egg yolk** also contains **unsaturated and polyun-**

---

15 Handelman et al., 1999

saturated FAs (oleic and linolenic acids) and **cholesterol (about 200 mg/egg).**

The "dark side" of eggs is their high cholesterol content. The daily requirement for cholesterol is estimated to be about 300 mg/day, and the guidelines suggest 2–4 medium eggs/week. Remember that bodily response to egg consumption varies among individuals and that dietary cholesterol is not the principal factor affecting circulating cholesterol levels, but also the intake of saturated and *trans*-FAs.[16]

---

16 Howell et al., 1997

DO's and DON'Ts

Having trouble getting the right daily dose of good protein? To make it easier, I've summarized the key points into some DO's and DON'Ts/LIMITs:

DO'S

1. **DO** be conscious about your protein intake. Get an idea of how much you should be eating daily according to gender, age, and physical activity, and try to divide wisely between your meals.
2. **DO** eat good protein, balancing between animal and vegetable protein.
3. **DO** look to get at least half of your daily protein requirement from legumes, whole grains, nuts, and vegetables such as broccoli, cauliflower, asparagus, green peas, Brussels sprouts, and spinach.
4. **DO** eat seafood; seafood is a great source of protein as well as omega-3 FAs.
5. **DO** eat poultry, better without the skin.
6. **DO** eat eggs. Eggs are rich in protein (egg white), cholesterol (egg yolk) and many vitamins.

DON'TS/LIMITS

1. **LIMIT** the amount of red meat and choose the leanest cuts, because red meat can contain a lot of saturated FAs.
2. **LIMIT** yourself to only very rarely eating processed meat.
3. **DON'T** forget dairy; despite its bad rap, dairy has a wealth of health benefits in appropriate quantities.

SUMMARY

Why eat protein?

Protein are the literal building blocks of life; what more need be said?

What and how much protein should we eat?

Protein should be 15–20 percent **of our daily caloric intake,** with **vegetable protein being the main source,** followed by **fish, meat, eggs and dairy.**

Our daily protein intake should be **0.8–1g per kg of weight a day for adults, and 1.2g per kg a day for the elderly** to counteract sarcopenia, a disease associated with the aging process which causes loss of muscle mass and strength.

	Serving Size	**Frequency**
Legumes serving	Fresh: 5–6 oz (140–170 g) Dried: 2.5–3 oz (70–80 g)	3 times/week
Fish serving	5–6 oz (140–170 g)	2–3 times/week
Meat serving: red meat	3.5–4 (100–110 g)	1 time/week
Poultry	4–5 oz (110–140 g)	2 times/week
Cold cuts	1.8 oz (50 g)	1 time or less/week
Milk	½–1 cup (120–240 ml)	Per day

	Serving Size	Frequency
Yogurt	½–1 cup (120–240 ml)	Per day
Cheese	2.5–3.5 oz (70–100 g)	1–2 times/week
Eggs	2–4 medium eggs	1 week

When during the day should we eat protein?

Each meal should include a certain amount of protein to cover the daily intake. However, the amount of protein at dinner should be higher than at lunch.

CHAPTER 7

Salt and the Mamma Mia! Diet

PASS THE SALT, PLEASE! In my grandparents' generation, this simple question was perfectly fine. However, in just a few generations, our salt consumption has reached toxic levels. And this is true for almost every culture and cuisine. In fact, I usually **do not put salt on the table** simply because salt is already present in all the food we eat, in particular in processed foods. The food industry adds salt like it's a magical substance, and there's reason to believe they're right: salt reduces bitterness, enhances sweetness, boosts flavor, and preserves perishable foods. And it's been this way for centuries; the use of salt in cooking dates back to ancient times, when our ancestors discovered that it could enhance the flavors of dishes and could be used to preserve foods. It was so important and precious that the ancient Romans built the *Via Salaria*, or the "salt road," to supply Rome with salt from the Adriatic Sea. Even the word "salary," the payment one receives from an employer in return for work performed, comes from the word salt; early Roman soldiers would receive some or all of their pay in the form of salt.

Put simply, salt has long been the engine behind empires and revolutions. And today, there's a new battle in the salt wars: on one side, we have the desire to produce foods that are tasty, cheap, and have a long shelf-life; on the other, the fight to shrink our waistline, lower our blood pressure and reduce our risk of other lifestyle-related diseases linked to sodium consumption.

WHAT IS SALT?

The word salt is actually a chemistry term, referring to a combination of an acid and a base, which together are neutral and have a crystal formation. However, when we use the term "salt" in everyday situations, we're referring to one particular salt—the common table salt, sodium chloride (NaCl). At room temperature, sodium chloride is a crystalline solid, is colorless, and has a distinctive smell and flavor.

Unfortunately, common table salt barely resembles naturally occurring salt, as the processes of refining and bleaching depletes the precious substances contained within. Naturally occurring salt is more or less a balanced compound in structure; in addition to the sodium chloride, other compounds are present, too, including magnesium chloride, magnesium sulfate, calcium sulfate, sulfate potassium, calcium carbonate, bromine, and iodine. We also find traces of all other known minerals, such as boron, barium, silicon, fluorine, lithium … the list goes on. All of these are elements that allow our bodies to function optimally.

But with industrial processing, salt is chemically cleaned and reduced to be just sodium chloride, with about 95 percent of the minerals and essential trace elements removed, considered as they are to be 'impurities' in the salt. Even sea salt or rock salt from a natural origin, which some may consider healthier, is put through an extensive "cleaning" process due to strict food safety regulations.

TABLE SALT: THE GOOD, THE BAD AND THE UGLY

The Good: Sodium is Necessary for Survival

Sodium chloride is essential for life. It is present in all bodily tissues and fluid, albeit in small amounts. Sodium facilitates the transmission of sensory and motor signals along nerves and aids in the absorption of some nutrients from our food. Chloride facilitates the balance of acid in the body and the absorption of potassium. But perhaps the most important role of salt is the regulation of hydration in our cells. An aqueous solution containing 0.9 percent sodium chloride is called a "physiological solution" because it has the same osmotic pressure as human blood plasma, and is therefore used in medicine to treat dehydration in cases where simple water is not sufficient.

Finally, salt can be prescribed to treat or prevent certain diseases. For example, iodized salt prevents and treats hypothyroidism, and potassium chloride can be used instead of sodium chloride for improving hypertension (with little change to flavor).

The Bad: The Health Consequences

So what if I eat too much salt, I hear you say. I'm not overweight and I eat healthily!

Like everything, the dose makes the poison. Consumption of sodium above the amount necessary for bodily functions has a direct and proven association with hypertension, or high blood pressure, which in turn leads to heart disease, stroke, obesity, and even type 2 diabetes. As sodium retains liquid, it has also been implicated in cellulitis which, although genetic and only cosmetic, is a marker of hydration. Food rich in salt, like processed meat, has even been associated with increased incidence of stomach cancer.[1] Too much salt also increases the urinary excretion of calcium, leading to osteoporosis.

Ask yourself: are you already at risk for any of the conditions mentioned? Do you have a family history of these diseases? Sodium has been linked to so many preventable diseases that it's not surprising the government spends billions on campaigning against it. Behind nearly every lifestyle-related, preventable disease, the ill effects of sodium overconsumption can be found. Its effects have touched the lives of nearly every human on this planet.

There is one simple mechanism which links all these diseases to sodium: **systemic inflammation**, or inflammation of the entire body. Sodium is implicated in systemic inflammation via hypertension and water retention, and has a flow of effect to these other diseases.

If you're looking to counteract some of the effects of the sodium imbued into all our food, consider the benefits of potassium. Modern people consume **too much salt and too little potassium**. In the case of high blood pressure, potassium reportedly counteracts the work of sodium. Potassium-rich foods include fruits and vegetables such as bananas, apricots, pears, tomatoes and avocado. Research is currently being conducted to confirm whether we can replace a percentage of our table salt with potassium chloride, which so far has shown promising results.

The Ugly: Our Sodium Reality

The World Health Organization (WHO) recommends an absolute maximum daily intake of 2.3 g of sodium (equal to one teaspoon of salt), though ideally, they'd like us to limit our intake to 1.5 g a day. Take out your salt shaker: this is equivalent to two thirds of a

---

1   Fang et al., 2015

teaspoon. Yet even after years of campaigning, Americans continue to consume (on average) around 4 g a day, with averages of over 9 g a day reported in some states.

Interestingly, a mere 10 percent of sodium consumed by Americans is inherent to the fresh food we eat, naturally occurring in fruit, vegetables, meat and dairy products. This constitutes the amount which we actually need, by the way. Another 5 percent of sodium intake is from salt added during cooking and food preparation; a further 6 percent is added at the table. If we stopped here, Americans would be consuming just 21 percent of the current average; in other words, they'd be within the recommended limit.

The remainder, a whopping **78 percent of sodium intake**, comes from processed foods. This includes sodium added when food products are "created," in processed products such as bread, crackers, cold cuts, cheese, canned foods, chips, and snacks. Salt is even added to sweet industrial products, such as cakes, cookies, breakfast cereals, and snack foods. Read the food labels; you will probably be surprised by how much salt you eat in a day. Some of the biggest secret offenders are bread, processed meat, and cheese, so if you make yourself a ham and cheese sandwich, chances are you've already gone over the daily limit!

USING SALT THE SMART WAY

Before anyone veers off to the other extreme, there's no need to swear off salt for life! As we have already discussed, there are definitely benefits to correct sodium intake. In ordinary kitchens, the use of salt primarily serves to enhance the flavor of foods. For this reason, it is used in basically all traditions and cuisines from around the world. Salt is still the key to the success of many dishes; we just need to think carefully about *how* we use the salt when preparing food.

To cook tasty yet nutritious dishes, it is important to add salt **at the right time**. Boiling vegetables in salted water keeps colors vivid and prevents the loss of vitamins and minerals (except for legumes). However, it is better to add your salt only a few minutes before removing legumes from the heat to keep them from becoming tough. If you cook meat, fish, eggs, and vegetables in a pan or in the oven, it is better to add salt towards the end of cooking, because salt can dry out the food while cooking and make it makes lose water.

IODIZED SALT

Iodized salt refers to refined salt which has small amounts of iodine added to it. Note the paradox: the salt manufacturing industry adds iodine to the refined salt, from which natural iodine was previously removed. They fortify the salt in this way because the world's population at large has a tendency to consume insufficient volumes of iodine to prevent thyroid disease by iodine deficiency, and salt is so over-consumed that it makes for the ideal delivery vehicle for such a fortification program.

However, consuming sea salt in its unrefined form will still provide you with some iodine, as well as a range of other minerals, too, so iodized salt should not be viewed as the "better alternative" to common table salt.

DOs and DON'Ts/LIMITs

Here are eight simple rules you can adopt to reduce your salt intake. Trust me; your health will thank you!

DO's

1. **DO** re-train your palate to prefer **less salt**. If you don't like the lack of flavor, remember this is normal; just reduce the salt content gradually.

2. **DO** use more **spices and herbs** to keep your dishes tasty. Chili, pepper, saffron, ginger, garlic, onion, thyme, basil, rosemary, or sage are excellent because they are sources of antioxidants and bioactive compounds.

3. **DO** use lemon juice and vinegar in place of salt. Both are enhancers of flavors. Like herbs and spices, their use allows us to reduce the amount of salt. Lemon also increases the availability of iron in vegetables; it is useful, for example, to season spinach with lemon.

4. **DO** be sure to always **ask for salt on the side** when eating out, only to be added by you as necessary.

5. **DO** measure your salt into the palm of your hand before putting it on your food so you can visually see how much salt you're adding. Remember to aim for not more than 1.7 g of sodium a day (equal to **3/4 of one teaspoon**). Don't aimlessly shake the shaker over your plate; the volume that comes out is deceptive!

6. **DO** learn which **foods have a "secret" sodium component**. These include breads, cereals, cheese, and just about any highly processed food. Read food labels to measure your sodium intake, and adapt your tastes to prefer the lower sodium options available.

DON'Ts/LIMITs

1. **DON'T** eat canned foods and foods preserved in salt without **carefully rinsing them** under cold running water to reduce salt content. Even better, opt for foods preserved in olive oil instead.
2. **LIMIT** the amount of canned fish preserved in brine, because it contains more salt than that preserved in olive oil.
3. **LIMIT** the amount of fast food, processed foods, and sauces such as ketchup, soy sauce, and mustard.
4. **DON'T** add salt to a baby's food, at the least not until they are one year old. Not only do you risk them adopting a salty palate, but their kidneys cannot yet handle much sodium.

SUMMARY

Why eat salt?

Sodium chloride *is* essential for life, and facilitates any number of bodily functions, including the regulation of hydration in our cells.

What and how much salt should we eat?

The World Health Organization (WHO) recommends an absolute maximum daily intake of 2.3 g of sodium (though ideally, they'd like us to limit our intake to 1.5 g a day), or about 2/3 of a teaspoon. You should look for salts that haven't been robbed of their natural benefits through a chemical purification process.

When should we eat salt?

Generally, it's best to make your salt intake a part of a recipe, as opposed to a seasoning after the fact. Boiling vegetables in salted water or adding a small amount of salt towards the end of cooking leads to flavorful dishes that will fulfill your daily salt requirement.

CHAPTER 8

Beverages and the Mamma Mia! Diet

I T SHOULD GO WITHOUT saying that what we drink is as just important as what we eat. Choosing the right drinks can improve the quality of our lives drastically, both by decreasing the risk of lifestyle related diseases and helping us maintain a healthy body weight. Many people drink large quantities of fluids that are full of empty calories and chemicals and with no nutritional value whatsoever. Others simply don't drink *enough* fluids.

WATER: THE ELIXIR OF LIFE

Water, one of the most important substances on earth, should be always be **fluid number one** in our diet. In humans, about 50–60 percent of our body weight is made up by **water;** for this reason, water is classified as an **essential nutrient** just like carbohydrates, lipids, protein, vitamins, and minerals. Water is involved in basically all bodily functions, including regulation of body temperature, transport of nutrients and other substances in the circulatory system, and delivery of essential minerals. It is also the vehicle used to eliminate waste products and toxins and provides structural support to tissues and joints. About 1½–2 quarts (1.5–2 liters) of water are lost each day through urine, sweat, and respiration, and since there is no efficient mechanism of water storage in the human body, a constant supply of fluid is needed to preserve water content. Our fluid needs can be partially satisfied by water contained in food we consume (vegetables and fruits), but a daily intake of 1– 1 ½ quarts (1–1.5 liters) of water is still needed.

Good hydration is essential for maintaining our body's water "*equilibrium*," although needs may vary among people depending on age, physical activity level, personal circumstances, and weather conditions. Adequate water intake, and especially that of natural mineral water, has been associated with a higher diet quality. Our Mamma Mia Diet guidelines suggest starting the day with a glass of warm water with lemon juice (unless you have gastric problems) so that your body can replace some of the fluids lost overnight and your kidney filtration capacity will be off to a great start.

There are many sources of water available, such as surface water, aquifer water, spring water, and seawater. An interesting source of water that has been recently studied is **deep sea water (DSW)**, which has been shown to be potentially beneficial as it can supply minerals that are essential to health. DSW commonly refers to seawater that is pumped up from a depth of over 650 feet (200 meters), where there is less photosynthesis of plant plankton, lower consumption of nutrients, and lots of organic decomposition, causing abundant nutrients to remain there. Research has demonstrated that DSW may help overcome lifestyle-associated diseases such as cardiovascular disease, diabetes, obesity, cancer, and skin problems.[1]

---

1 Samihah Zura Mohd Nani et al., 2016

WHY RED WINE IS GREAT—AND GREAT FOR YOU

Wine has been an intrinsic part of Italian culture for centuries. In fact, if you ask Italians, they're likely say that wine is almost as important as the food in an Italian meal. Wine is a pleasure of life that dates back to ancient times. The origin of wine actually lies in ancient Mesopotamia, sometime between 4,000 and 3,000 BCE. The Greeks brought the art of winemaking to southern Italy and Sicily; the Etruscans, hailing from Asia Minor, later introduced it to central Italy. The Romans enjoyed wine very much, and made some important improvements in how it is produced. They enhanced the Greek presses used for extracting the juices from grapes, increasing the yields, which became especially important as the demand for wine grew with population expansion.

Today, Italian wine is one of our country most well-known exports. In 2016, the International Organization of Vine and Wine estimated that Italy was the largest wine producer worldwide. Part of this is due to Italy having many diverse wine regions, corresponding to different climates. Understanding Italian wine becomes easier with an understanding of the differences between each region, whose cuisine reflects the indigenous wines and vice versa.

Wine is made from water, pressed grapes, and yeast, which is fermented and then aged in oak barrels. The finished product contains **ethanol** (alcohol), natural **sugars** (glycerol and polysaccharides), and different types of bioactive molecules such as **flavonols** (which include quercetin), **flavones**, **anthocyanidins**, **stilbenes** (and its derivate, resveratrol), and **tannins**. The right combination of grape variety, environment of the vineyard, aging, barrel composition, and balance of bioactive molecules produced during fermentation all make Italian wines tasty, healthy, and special.

In Italy, we say, "*Il vino rosso fa buon sangue*," meaning, "*Red wine makes good blood.*" This is a simple way to say that red wine keeps you healthy.

In most countries, high intake of saturated fat correlates to high mortality rates from coronary heart disease (CHD). In France, however, the rule seems not to hold; in fact, the high intake of saturated fat is concurrent with *low* mortality from CHD. This paradox is explained in part by moderate consumption of red wine.[2] Additionally, a large number of studies have demonstrated that wine intake may have a beneficial effect on mortality.[3] In fact, the alcohol component in wine (ethanol) increases HDL cholesterol levels, inhibits platelet aggregation, and reduces systemic inflammation.

Sufficient evidence exists which supports a **significant inverse association between regular and moderate wine consumption and vascular risk**, particularly red wine, and a similar relationship is reported for beer consumption, while lower protection is described for the consumption of spirits.[4]

The Health Benefits of Red Wine

Additional benefits of red wine—compared to those of other alcoholic beverages—are probably due to its higher polyphenolic content, which has been shown to **modulate platelet aggregation, cellular redox state, and carbohydrate and lipid metabolism**.[5] **Resveratrol** is a type of antioxidant naturally found in grape skins and red grape juice. Unlike white wine, red wine is fermented on the skins, which changes its properties drastically. White wine is also made from grapes, but the grapes are pressed and only the juice is fermented, discarding the skins completely, so it is not such a good source of resveratrol. Curiously, resveratrol is absorbed only when is ingested from wine,[6] and it is likely that the beneficial effects may

---

2 Renaud and de Lorgeril, 1992
3 Grønbaek et al., 2000
4 Arteroa et al., 2015
5 Arteroa et al., 2015
6 Bertelli, 2005

be attributed to the overall mix of all its components. The reason for this appears to be the requirement for a particular matrix in which resveratrol works in synergy with other biocompounds.[7]

Wine provides 7 calories per gram, and the recommended limits are 1½ glasses a day for women, and 2 glasses a day for men. A glass of wine is equal to ½ cup, or 120 ml. Wine should be consumed during meal and never on an empty stomach.

The health benefits associated with the Mamma Mia Diet, which combines moderate wine consumption with a diet rich in fruits, vegetables, legumes, whole grains, fish, and extra virgin olive oil, suggests that polyphenols have synergistic effects with compounds found in other groups of foods. Very importantly, wine consumption should not replace a healthy lifestyle, but it can be part of it.

GUIDELINES FOR OTHER TYPES OF ALCOHOL

Moderate alcohol consumption is defined in the Dietary Guidelines for Americans (2010) as up to 1 drink per day for women and up to 1½ drinks per day for men. The Mamma Mia Diet advises you to limit your consumption of other types of alcohol (not wine) to seldom, if at all. In addition, you shouldn't add to your daily wine consumption.

Alcohol abuse or **binge drinking** is linked to a large number of medical, social, and work-related problems, including the development of **alcohol dependence syndrome**, several chronic diseases, such as liver cirrhosis, cardiomyopathy, encephalopathies, polyneuropathy, and dementia, and accidents which eventually lead to death.

There is extensive evidence that **alcohol abuse increases the risk of developing cancer of the oral cavity, pharynx, larynx, esophagus, and liver.** In 2007, the International Agency for Research on

---

7 Gertsch, 2011

Cancer and the World Cancer Research Fund/American Institute for Cancer Research stated that alcohol also increases the risk for **colon, rectal, and breast cancer.**[8]

JUICE: FRESH-SQUEEZED VS PRE-PACKAGED

Don't judge a juice by its carton! Or rather, do; just read the label on the packaging, and I can promise you'll be back to the old-style homemade freshly squeezed juice before you know it.

I, along with many other Italians, love to order a *spremuta d'arancia* (freshly squeezed orange juice) along with their breakfast in the "*bar.*" Drinking a glass of freshly squeezed juice in the morning is not only delicious, but provides numerous health benefits such as better retention of vitamins, minerals, enzymes, and antioxidants—all of which gets lost in the processing that juices in bottles or cartons undergo.

Drinking freshly squeezed juice can also be an efficient way to reach the recommended daily servings of fruits and vegetables, as well as to bump up water consumption. Juices are easily absorbed by the body because the nutrients from fruits and vegetables are already broken down by the juicer into a digestible form that the body can easily use. When you juice fruits or vegetables, remember to add 2 tablespoons of the pulp left in the juicer back into your glass; it's these solid parts that contain the food's fiber.

As soon as you juice your fruits or vegetables, you are breaking down the cell walls, thereby activating all the vitamins, enzymes and phytonutrients found in the food. Therefore, it is recommended to drink juices as soon as they are prepared.

Fresh juices contain natural sugars, but the amounts are much smaller than in processed juices, which contain many other added

---

8 IARC Working Group on the Evaluation of Carcinogenic Risks to Humans, 2010

ingredients, such as fructose, corn syrup, and food coloring—all substances that do not provide any real nutritional value to our body. (You can read more extensively about the differences in Chapter 3: Carbohydrates and the Mamma Mia! Diet.)

When reading the packaging and labels of processed juices, be alert for terms like "from concentrate," "juice drink," "juice blend," or "juice cocktail." These are not the healthy drinks that you would want to add to your diet—these products are often made using a blend of syrup, sugar, flavoring, coloring, and water, and never taste as refreshing as fresh juice. Instead, look for "freshly squeezed" or "made from freshly squeezed" when making your purchase.

SOFT DRINKS

Soft drinks have no place in the Mamma Mia Diet—period. Without exception, you are better off avoiding them. In the last century, the popularity of soft drinks has exploded internationally, mostly due to availability. They are available at any time of day in all sorts of locations; they're cheap; and they have a long shelf life—not to mention that advertising for soft drinks is forced upon us from a young age.

A soft drink is a drink that typically contains no alcohol (hence the name *soft*), carbonated water, large amounts of sugars (mostly high fructose corn syrup) or artificial sweeteners (aspartame or sucralose, which I'll talk about next), flavoring (usually phosphoric acid, which gives a tangy taste in the mouth, and citric acid), and caffeine (though some drinks are decaffeinated). Although typically sweet, soda and soft drinks are not so sweet as to stop people consuming these drinks alongside their meals. Despite this, soda generally contains a whopping 10–13 of your daily sugar requirement—clearly junk food material.

A soft drink contains a lot of calories—empty calories—and no nutrients, which means it doesn't contribute in any way to helping our body function. And isn't that the definition of food—matter which we consume in order to nourish our body so it can perform certain functions? There's some food for thought. (For more information on sugar and sweeteners, refer to Chapter 4: Carbohydrates and the Mamma Mia Diet.)

Diet soft drinks, which contain no calories (and no nutrients, remember) instead contain artificial sweeteners. These are technically also sugars, but are manufactured in a laboratory so that they have an excessively sweet taste compared to natural sugar. This means that only tiny volumes are required to achieve a sweet taste. A common concern with artificial sweeteners is that the safety and consequences of consuming large amounts is unknown because these substances are so new to the human diet, so no long-term studies are available yet. In addition, those who *can* afford to run such clinical trials may be biased; for example, studies may be conducted or funded by food industry giants.

Soft drinks also contain phosphoric acid, which can act as a flavoring and preservative, keeping the contents of the bottle or can fresh. Several studies found that drinking just four cans of regular or diet Coca-Cola a week led to lower bone density in women—a condition that increases the risk of osteoporosis. And in fact, soft drinks have long been implicated in lower calcium levels and higher phosphoric acid levels in the blood. When phosphoric acid levels are high and calcium levels are low, calcium is pulled out of the bones to compensate. Since the phosphoric acid content of soft drinks is very high and they contain virtually no calcium, calcium is displaced from bones by the phosphoric acid, lowering the bone density of the skeleton and leading to weakened bones. Making things worse, when amounts of phosphoric acid are in excess, the kidneys have a reduced capacity to excrete it. So what happens is that soft drinks remove calcium from the bones and deposit it in the kidney, which is too overworked to excrete it, resulting in kidney stones. Research has shown that phosphoric acid can accelerate aging,[9] and that a low calcium-to-phosphorus ratio in the diet increases the incidence of hypertension and the risk of colorectal cancer.

There is accumulating evidence supporting a link between sugar-sweetened beverages and a number of health problems. The spike in energy is likely to be a major contributor to **weight gain and increased risk of type 2 diabetes.**[10]

The bottom line? The Mamma Mia Diet advises you drink fewer soft drinks, diet drinks, and pre-packaged juices and replace them with water, fresh juices, green tea, or herbal tea. This is a healthier habit for general health, as well as weight control.

THE COFFEE CONTROVERSY

The debate over the impact of coffee on our health has been controversial. There have been more than 30,000 studies worldwide, without any conclusive results. One thing is certain, however; the response to coffee—and especially to caffeine, the alcaloid present in coffee—varies greatly from person to person. For example, some people drink coffee in the evening and sleep well; others cannot sleep at all. I usually do not drink coffee in evening; I prefer my cappuccino in the morning!

Caffeine content varies by size of the drinking cup, bean origin, roasting, and preparation methods.

Coffee is produced by the plant Coffea, whose seeds, called coffee beans, are used to make various coffee beverages and products. The history of coffee goes at least as far back as the 10th century in Africa (Ethiopia). By the 16th century, coffee had reached the Middle East, India, Turkey, and northern Africa, before spreading to the Balkans, Italy, and finally America. While it may have been the

---

9 Ohnishi and Razzaque, 2010
10 Helm and Macdonald, 2015

Arabs and the Turks who brought coffee to Italy, it is the Italians who made drinking coffee an art.

Coffee *is* a pleasure of life, but, like anything, moderation is the key. Two coffees a day are certainly a treat we should not be forced to give up; especially in Italy, where coffee is not only a drink, but a ritual engrained deep into our culture. The art of preparing and drinking coffee in Italy is comparable to the tea ceremony in Japan, though it is not such a time-consuming activity. In fact, we take only a few minutes to drink it, not even sitting down, but standing at the counter in the café.

Coffee is certainly a form of socialization: no matter the time or the day, it is always an opportunity to spend time together with friends. "*Andiamo a prendere un caffè,*" "Let's go and have a coffee," is a common suggestion in Italy. Having coffee together means enjoying a break during the day and sharing more than just time with colleagues and friends. Coffee is certainly a form of socialization: no matter the time or the day, it is always an opportunity to spend time together with friends.

Espresso, which is coffee brewed by forcing a small amount of nearly boiling water (200°F or 93°C) under pressure through finely ground coffee beans, is generally thicker than coffee brewed by other methods, is richer in aroma, can be enjoyed in particular after eating a meal, and can help with digestion. It is also the base for other drinks such as *cappuccino, latte macchiato* (flat white, or latte in English), *caffè macchiato* (espresso with a small amount of milk), or delicious desserts like the well-known *tiramisù* (which literally translates to a pick-me-up). Italians drink espresso all day long, but have a specific time for *cappuccino* and *latte macchiato*. Such milky coffees, heavier than a simple espresso, are for breakfast, and never after a meal or late in the afternoon.

An Italian coffee is certainly healthier than American coffee. Concoctions rich in sugar or flavored using artificial syrups or powders would never be found in an Italian café. An espresso, taken without milk, does not have any calories at all, and may contribute to weight loss because it contains caffeine. **Black coffee,** coffee without milk or sugar, is not only tasty but contains a number of micronutrients, notably potassium, magnesium, and niacin or vitamin B3. The type of water used in preparation (for example, hard or soft water) may influence the micronutrient content of a cup of black coffee, particularly in relation to calcium and magnesium levels. Slight variations in composition may occur due to origin, growing conditions, blend composition, and processing of the coffee.

Caffeine, which is also found in tea, soft drinks, chocolate and energy drinks, has an effect on the body's metabolism and therefore its energy expenditure. Caffeine stimulates the central nervous system, which can make you feel more alert and give you a boost of energy (though in excessive amounts, it has undesirable effects on anxiety). Some people are more sensitive to the effects of caffeine than others, and studies have demonstrated that people who have more than 2–3 coffees per day can acquire a physical dependence that triggers withdrawal symptoms including headaches, muscle pain and stiffness, lethargy, nausea, vomiting, depressed mood, and marked irritability. Although espresso has more caffeine per unit volume than most coffee beverages, this is only because the portion size is smaller than an American cup, so the actual concentration of caffeine consumed is much lower.

Scientific evidence has shown that coffee may protect from age-related diseases such as Alzheimer's and Parkinson's[11] through the activation of protein Nrf2, a switch for antioxidative proteins. In fact, free radicals seem to play an important role in these age-related diseases. Coffee's role in cancer protection is mixed; it may protect from some types of cancers, but may also increase the risk of stomach cancer. Many of the compounds in coffee, like caffeine and the various acidic compounds found in coffee beans, can irritate the stomach and the lining of small intestine. It is known to be a

11 Chen et al., 2010

problem for those suffering from ulcers, gastritis, IBS, and Crohn's disease; doctors generally advise patients with these conditions to avoid coffee completely. This is one reason why we should not drink coffee on an empty stomach. In conclusion, we can say that recent scientific information has generated a new concept of coffee, which does not match the common belief that coffee is mostly harmful. Coffee—in moderation—can actually be beneficial.[12]

THE DANGERS OF ENERGY DRINKS

Energy drinks are advertised to increase energy, physical performance, and even intellectual prowess. They differ in typical ingredients, but most of them include high doses of caffeine, sugar, vitamins, and **controversial** ingredients such as **guarana, ginseng, and taurine**. A recent study has demonstrated that the consumption of energy drinks increases performance in muscle strength and endurance exercises, with performance correlated with the quantity of taurine.[13] But more recently, strong controversy has surrounded the possible adverse effects of excessive consumption of energy drinks, associated with high caffeine consumption. The quantity of caffeine in a typical energy drink is about 80–160 mg per serving, and both the American and European food authorities (US FDA and EFSA) believe that the maximum daily limit of caffeine for an adult, in order to avoid adverse health effects, is about 400 mg per day (300 mg for adolescents and pregnant women).

There is accumulating evidence that overconsumption of energy drinks in adolescents, especially when consumed before or during sports practice, may trigger a number of atypical disorders for this age, including heart palpitations, arrhythmia, anxiety, nausea, heart attacks, and even sudden death.[14] Lastly, although the effects

12Cano-Marquina et al., 2013
13 Souza et al., 2017
14 Sanchis-Gomar et al., 2016

of caffeine consumption on brain development have not yet been examined, it is hypothesized that caffeine may alter normal brain development during critical developmental periods. It is even theorized that energy drinks abuse by young adolescents predicts the use of legal and illegal substances later in life.[15]

In recent years, a particular *"dangerous liaison"* has become popular among adolescents: **alcohol mixed with energy drinks**. A growing body of studies show a link between the use of alcoholic energy drinks and increased impulsivity, which in turn leads to an overconsumption of alcohol and an enhanced desire to drink more, compared to alcohol alone, increasing the risk of developing addictive behaviors.[16] Adolescents consuming both alcohol and energy drinks are at a **higher risk of negative behavioral outcomes;** recently, Dr. Van Rjin was quoted as saying, "Drinking highly caffeinated alcoholic beverages triggers changes in the adolescent brain **similar to taking cocaine**, and the consequences last into adulthood as an altered ability to deal with rewarding substances."[17] For these reasons, the FDA has determined that caffeine is an unsafe food additive when combined with alcohol.

Put simply, consumption of energy drinks is not recommended. Above all, it is strongly advised that energy drinks not be offered to children, and it is extremely dangerous to consume energy drinks containing alcohol.

15 Barrense-Dias, 2016
16 Rossheim et al., 2016; Lalanne et al., 2107
17 Robins et al., 2016

DO's and DON'Ts

Having a hard time getting the right daily dose of fluids? Struggling to avoid temptation, displacing water consumption with nasty alternatives? To make things easier I've summarized things into some DO's and DON'Ts/LIMITs:

DO'S
1. **DO** drink plenty of natural water, about 1–1½ quarts (or 1–1.5 liters) a day.
2. **DO** drink freshly squeezed fruit or vegetable juice, adding two tablespoons of the remaining pulp left behind in the juicer. Consume 1–2 glasses a day.
3. **DO** drink good red wine, up to 1½ glasses a day for women, and 2½ glasses a day for men during meals, though not on an empty stomach.
4. **DO** drink coffee. You can have up to two coffees a day of your favorite type of coffee, though not on an empty stomach.

DON'TS/LIMITS
1. **DON'T** drink soft drinks or energy drinks—ever.
2. **LIMIT** consumption of alcohol (other than wine) to 1 drink a day for women and up to 1 ½ drinks a day for men.

SUMMARY

What should we be drinking?

The majority of our hydration should, of course, come from clean water. Fresh-squeezed fruit juice and vegetable juice is also recommended. Things like sugary beverages, alcoholic mixed drinks and energy drinks are not suitable, and carry a host of health risks. However, a glass or two of good red wine can be healthy and is a part of the traditional Mediterranean diet.

When should we be drinking?

Water consumption should occur throughout the day; keeping our body hydrated is key to staying energized and motivated, and making sure all of our body's processes work properly.

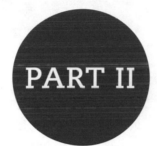

PART II

Top Tips for Success

CHAPTER 9

Shop Intelligently

G OOD NUTRITION STARTS WITH smart shopping. By stocking our shelves with only the healthiest ingredients and foods, we remove the temptation to eat poorly and give ourselves every resource necessary to maintain a healthy, supportive diet.

While it may seem difficult to fit shopping into our busy schedules, the fact is that we can learn how to shop with pleasure, dedicating time to ourselves and our family. This time is an investment in an improved lifestyle, and all it requires is a certain degree of planning.

So, how should you learn to shop intelligently? It easier than it sounds; here are some of the rules I follow which, once you adopt them, will make your shopping experience quicker, easier, and healthier!

Make a shopping list of what you actually need for the week.

My suggestion is to plan your meals out in advance, make a list of what you'll need, and buy only the ingredients on the list, avoiding junk and processed food. The risk of shopping without a list is that you will buy too much food, make impulse purchases (usually of junk food), and leave yourself with temptation at home. Don't underestimate the appeal of the food in your own cupboards—it is very hard to say no to food you've already purchased! Shopping lists also help with meal planning (refer to Chapter 10: Meal Patterns and Planning); if you have a list, you're less likely to make poor, last-minute choices such as takeout or frozen meals.

Don't shop when you're hungry.

Your eyes are bigger than your stomach, and much less trustworthy! Don't be tempted by unplanned choices.

Try to shop more at the local farmers' market.

There's nothing I love more than shopping at the farmers' market in my own town of Como, Italy. Where else can I pick up fresh, seasonal fruits and vegetables, local cheeses, and organic meat from my local area? I love to go there early in the morning when the farmers display all their products, talking to them and tasting the new arrivals. This allows me to develop a relationship with the people I buy from.

In addition, shopping at local markets promotes the zero-kilometer food movement, which encourages consumption of food from your local region which hasn't been imported from abroad and hasn't travelled for hours (or sometimes days) in a truck. This means the food the consumers receive is fresher, and so hasn't had the opportunity to lose nutrients (which starts from the moment of harvest). It supports local economies, promotes sustainability, and helps reduce carbon emissions, too! If you make this a life-long habit, food shopping will become an opportunity to socialize; it will become the "trip" of the day (and provide some physical activity, too).

Always read the labels.

The easiest rule to remember when reading food labels is simply to find foods that don't have a label at all! If they don't have a label, the food probably has just one ingredient—itself. The fewer ingredients there are on a label, the closer to the original source the food is. Remember to also check the amount of "good" and "bad" fat (refer to Chapter 5: Fat and the Mamma Mia! Diet), carbohydrates (it is obligatory in most countries for nutritional labels to contain both the total carbohydrate and sugar content), fiber, protein, vitamins, minerals, and sodium. As well as the overall calories, also check the calories per serving; for example, 40 calories per 3.5 oz (100 g) is considered low, 100 per 100 g is moderate, and 400 is high. Check that your serving size matches the one listed on the packet. Some words to avoid at all costs: *trans* fats, added sugar, sweetener, food coloring, and chemicals which don't provide any nutrition. Shop for real food; before buying a food product with a long list of ingredients, ask yourself if your grandmother would recognize it as food!

DON'T TRUST THE PACKAGING

Just because a product's packaging looks healthy and says that is healthy doesn't mean it is. Over many years, the food industry has created many substances that trigger our biochemistry to release hormones and enzymes at different rates, often increasing hunger, resulting in an increased risk of obesity, diabetes, cardiovascular disease, and some types of cancer. Our brain develops an addiction to these new changes as our taste buds change to adjust. These substances were created to make food cheaper, have a longer shelf-life, and to be tastier (usually using salt) than their natural counterparts, all of which earns companies more money. Don't let the food industry trick you—become a smart food detective and learn to read labels!

Check the preparation/expiration dates

It is obligatory for companies to list at least an expiration or "use by" date on packages. The longer the food sits on the supermarket shelves, the less fresh it is. Fresh food is always richer in nutrients and contains fewer preservatives. If it has a long shelf-life, this indicates that it is being preserved in some way, be it through preservatives, salt, vacuum-packaging, or oils.

Stop thinking that buying fresh and healthy food is more expensive.

We have been brainwashed by the food industry to believe that buying fresh food and cooking it at home is more expensive than buying pre-prepared, "inexpensive" fast food. Research has shown that eating real food is in fact **not more expensive**, and actually ends up **cheaper** in the long term, as it is an investment in our health. This is for several reasons; first, raw ingredients don't actually cost more because we aren't required to pay for packaging and preparation. Consider the price of fruits and vegetables per pound or kilogram: it's often very low. Second, the cost of advertising and running a large-scale business in incorporated into the price of prepared food, a cost which is universally passed on to the consumer. Finally, the cost of our health increases as we age, as lifestyle diseases such as obesity, heart disease, and diabetes begin to manifest as a result of accumulated bad habits over many years. If we do not take care of our health today, we will have to take care of our illness tomorrow.

MY WEEKLY SHOPPING LIST

The following is an example of my weekly shopping list, to give you an idea of what your shopping basket should look like when it comes time to check out!

	Percentage of basket	Percentage of budget
Whole grain cereals (pasta, bread, rice and other grains)	20%	10%
Fresh, local and seasonal fruits and vegetables	50%	10%
Good quality extra virgin olive oil	1–2%	5%
Legumes	5%	2%
Nuts	1–2%	2%
Fish	8%	32%
Eggs	1–2%	1–2%
Dairy products: milk, butter, fresh cheeses and Parmesan cheese	5%	5%
Meat (possibly organic, usually poultry over red meat)	5%	25%
Fresh herbs and spices	1–2%	1–2%
Honey, maple syrup, jam	1–2%	1–2%
Coffee and herb tea	1–2%	1–2%
Good quality wine	1–2%	5%

CHAPTER 10

Meal Patterns
and Planning

ODAY, OUR EATING PATTERNS are increasingly varied. Typical meals patterns like **breakfast, lunch, and dinner—** the way I grew up—are not common anymore. Instead, skipping meals and consuming many smaller snacks is becoming more prevalent. Such eating habits can have various effects on our cardiometabolic markers, which have been reported to have adverse effects on obesity, lipid profile, insulin resistance, and blood pressure.[1]

WHAT IS MEAL PLANNING?

Meal planning is whatever we plan to prepare and consume, including all of our meals and snacks during the day, whether that's breakfast, lunch, or dinner. It is also the plan we make before we shop.

Meal planning is a truly personal thing. What works for one may not work for another person. The goal, in my opinion, is to find a process that is both enjoyable and efficient: efficient for time, for money, and certainly for health. These are some of my simple

---

1 St-Onge et al., 2017

rules: I try to stick to a simple plan according to my schedule that week—how many days I am at home for a full day, who will be home on which days, and how many meals I'll have with friends, either at home or out. Then, I divide my week into meals, keeping in mind that every day is different. You will get bored of eating the same food too often, and it is healthier to consume a wide variety of food, so a different menu for each day of the week is a valuable asset.

I usually have a vegetarian day once a week (usually on Monday, as over the weekend I occasionally indulge in heavier foods). Growing up in a Catholic family, we had meat-free Fridays in remembrance of the day that Jesus died on the cross; I still try to keep this tradition alive in my family by having fish on these days.

Over the weekend, I cook more elaborate dishes, which I enjoy with my family and friends, an action of love for the people I care for. If you have a quiet weekend or some extra time, weekends are also a good opportunity to prepare many dishes for the week that can easily be stored either in the refrigerator or in the freezer.

In the recipes section, I've selected four different seasonal menus that I particularly enjoy to give you an idea of how to prepare an Italian menu according to the MMD year-round.

UNDERSTANDING MEAL PATTERNS

Our metabolism (which includes our appetite, digestion and the breakdown of macronutrients) is influenced by the dark/light cycle, following circadian rhythms. **Circadian rhythms** in our body are controlled by a central clock in the hypothalamus, as well as by clocks in peripheral organs like the intestine and the liver. We digest meals better during the day, when the body is efficient; whereas at night, the liver and the intestine slow down their functions while we sleep, and the breakdown of cholesterol and management of glucose is less effective. When we choose to eat, and the resulting efficiency of digestion, can have cardiometabolic implications via alterations of these peripheral clocks. Studies have suggested that eating late at night or skipping breakfast may be associated with weight gain and obesity, whereas intermittent fasting and high meal frequency may have beneficial cardiometabolic health effects.[2] For example, in an Italian group of centenarians, it was observed that the common feature of a long and healthy life was the consumption of meals at a regular time every day, and a long period of fasting, which lasts 10–12 hours during the night.

How Many Meals a Day Should We Eat?

It is important never to skip the three main meals: breakfast, the most important meal of the day (the "king"); lunch (the "prince"); and dinner, (the "pauper"). We should also eat two light snacks throughout the day, one in the morning and the other in the afternoon. I usually snack on a piece of fresh fruit, a serving of yogurt (½ cup or 120 ml), or a few unsalted nuts. Remember: the Mamma Mia Diet says fast food does not need to be junk food!

BREAKFAST: THE MOST IMPORTANT MEAL OF THE DAY

It's true! **Breakfast is the most important meal of the day**. Eating a healthy breakfast provides the right nutrients and fuel we need to get through a busy morning. Our metabolisms don't immediately receive the message that it's go-time when we first wake up, like other organs do (such as the brain). To ensure we have sufficient energy for getting on with our day, it's important for our organs to be switched back on. Breakfast functions to kick-start our metabolism and then to subsequently curb our appetite throughout the day. Breakfast should provide the greatest proportion of energy out of all the meals, followed by lunch and then by dinner.

2 Hutchinson et Heilbronn, 2016

Many people feel they aren't hungry in the morning because the digestive system has been dormant for several hours, or because they had a rich dinner (or even worse, a midnight snack!) Other times it may seem tempting to get an extra ten minutes of sleep by not eating breakfast, but this will cost us in other ways. Have you ever felt a raging hunger mid-morning after skipping breakfast? Studies have shown that breakfast-skippers have poor concentration, more fatigue, and a less healthy body weight than those who eat in the morning. So, no, there is never an excuse for skipping breakfast!

A typical MMD breakfast means starting the day with a glass of warm water mixed with the juice of half a lemon. Warm water and lemon is a natural energizer and detoxifier: it hydrates *and* oxygenates the body. Before putting food in, it also helps slowly wake up the digestive system and produce a healthy bowel movement. Being Italian, I also cannot skip my morning **cappuccino**; it is my morning pleasure. Mediterranean cultures often start the day with **dark coffee or tea,** or even a cappuccino, according to taste.

Your breakfast should contain some carbohydrates, some protein and fruit:

- **Complex carbohydrates**, which give you a more sustained release of energy, should definitely be a part of your breakfast. For example, include **1–2 slices of whole grain bread** (see page 178 in Part III: Recipes and Seasonal Menus for a recipe to make your own) with 1–2 teaspoons of homemade jam (refer to the recipe on page 166); or other try an **unsweetened cereal** like one serving (½ cup or 70 g) of homemade muesli (refer to my *Homemade Muesli* recipe on page 168) or **oatmeal porridge** with **fruit, 2–3 nuts, and 1 teaspoon of seeds**.
- **Protein** for breakfast should come from **cow, nut, or soy milk** sources. Try **yogurt** such as Greek yogurt, about1 serving (½ cup or 120 ml); or **eggs** (1–2 eggs is equivalent to one serving).

- **Fruit** should be always present at breakfast. It is an excellent source of **vitamins, minerals, and fiber**. A piece of fresh fruit such as an apple, orange, or banana can be combined with your carbohydrates or protein, or eaten separately. In fact, the morning is the best time of the day to eat a bounty of fruit. Alternatively, you could have fruit as a mid-morning snack between breakfast and lunch. You may prefer to have a **fruit shake** (refer to *Paola's Peach Shake* on page 172) or some freshly squeezed fruit juice. Remember: when you squeeze fruit, remember to add two tablespoons of the remaining pulp left in the juicer, because the solid parts of fruit contain the fiber.

On the weekend, when you have more time, you can indulge in something more elaborate or requiring more time to prepare, like red rice pudding (refer to my *Rice Pudding* recipe on page 176) or a toast with poached egg and avocado (see *Sunday Breakfast* recipe on page 174).

LUNCH: THE "PRINCE" MEAL

Lunch is the second most important meal of the day—the "prince" of meals! It is your second opportunity to **maintain your energy levels,** giving you the fuel you need to keep going. A healthy lunch can give you the energy to stay focused and pay attention at work, at school, at the gym, or doing whatever is required for you in a day.

The quantity and quality of the food you eat is a function of your activity levels and the time available. Although nearly everybody eats lunch, it is important to take time out of your day to stop, prepare, and eat lunch calmly. Try to find at least a thirty-minute window in the day to devote to lunch. It would be ideal to start your meal with a salad (refer to *Starters* for ideas) dressed with ½–1 tablespoon of extra virgin olive oil, lemon juice, or a teaspoon of **balsamic vinegar** (and a pinch of salt, according to your taste; I do not add it). A few nuts or a teaspoon of seeds can be added to the salad, too. Salads are low in calories, high in fiber, and rich in vitamins and minerals. Fiber helps us feel full, making us eat less for the remaining meal. In addition, fiber decreases the GI of carbohydrates, so it's an ideal combination with a pasta dish. When you eat salad, **never limit your portion size!** You can eat as much as you feel like!

As a **main course at lunch**, Italians often enjoy a plate of **pasta**. One serving of pasta is equal to **2.5–3 oz (70–80 g)** and is accompanied by plenty of **vegetables** and some fish or cheese. Some days we substitute pasta with another type of grain, like rice, spelt, or barley, of which **one serving is equal to scarcely ½ cup (about 70–80 g, depending on the type of grain), with some vegetables and legumes**. The amount of grains may vary according to combinations with other ingredients.

When your main dish includes animal protein (for example, from meat or fish), it would be better to avoid a salad which includes cheese, because this combination slows down digestion.

DINNER: THE "PAUPER" MEAL

Dinner should be **nutritious but light**; better yet, dinner should not be rich in food that gives us energy, such as glucose. Because our bodies don't need that in the evening, it could be transformed into fat. Dinner should be the last meal of the day, meaning no snacking afterwards. Dinner should be ideally consumed early in the evening; I usually eat my dinner between 7:00–8:00 pm. It is important that you have time to digest the food before you go to bed. Evidence suggests that eating more calories later at night is associated with obesity.

Regarding content, you have to follow a similar pattern to that of lunch, but including a little more protein and a little less carbohydrates. You can start with a glass of water, plenty of salad, and, as a main course, some protein. Consume fish at least three times a week, and meat (preferably chicken) two to three times a week. A single serving size may vary from **4–6 oz (110–170 g),** depending on the food type, age, gender, and physical activity. As a side dish, try some sautéed vegetables and rice, such as basmati or brown rice (¼-½ cup or 45-70 g). Alternatively, depending on the season, you can enjoy a soup or a *frittata*, an Italian style omelet (refer to page 241).

I usually will enjoy an herbal tea after dinner (such as mint, ginger, fennel, aniseed, and licorice). Tea is relaxing, helps digestion, and prevents bloating.

PREPARING YOUR PLATE

When putting together your plate for lunch or dinner, **half of each plate** should be made up **of vegetables and some fruit**—the stars of the plate! Try starting with something raw, colorful, and full of flavor, such as a salad, before a meal. This adds fiber and helps control appetite. The rest can be made up using cooked vegetable dishes, using as much variety and color as possible to ensure you receive the widest range of micronutrients. You can consume a fruit either half an hour **before a meal, by itself, together with a starter, or else after the meal** as dessert. There is a lot of controversy about fruit consumption at mealtime. Learn to listen to your body. Some people find fruit consumption right after a large meal means too much food is being held in the stomach for too long, causing fullness and even bloating from fermentation.

The other half of the plate should be divided between protein and carbohydrates, of which whole grains are the better choice. The proportion of carbohydrates and protein may vary slightly between lunch and dinner—give more value to carbs at lunch and to protein at dinner. **Extra virgin olive oil** is the king of fats. Use it to reach your fat quota for your meal, together with plenty of spices and fresh herbs. Remember that salt should be consumed only in moderation; however, by consuming fresh foods and a very limited amount of packaged food products, you're already eliminating a huge amount of potential salt consumption, so you can allow yourself a pinch of salt on your salad or vegetables. **Drink plenty of water.** This means **1–1½ quarts (1–1.5 liters)** each day. A glass before each meal will help control appetite and aid digestion. You can also enjoy a glass of good quality red wine with your meal, remembering that the recommended limits are 1½ glasses per day for women and 2½ glasses per day for men.

MEAL PLANNING TIPS

Make Time for Mealtime

Whenever you can, take the time to sit down at the table and enjoy your meal, sharing it with your loved ones. This is the time of the day to connect with your family—that's conviviality! It is also a way to relieve the stress accumulated throughout the day, and it promotes a feeling of well-being. However, don't stay at the dinner table late into the evening. Even after the food has been consumed, just one other person snacking or offering extra portions encourages the whole family to get into bad habits of over-consumption. Spend an hour or so enjoying a meal together, then migrate together to the living room if you desire more socialization. Leave the food in the kitchen, and don't encourage mindless snacking in front of the TV. By sitting around the dinner table too long or by eating a meal or snack in the living room, we take our attention off our meal and risk eating until we reach a state of over-fullness, which is firstly unnecessary and secondly damages weight control.

Chewing Your Food

Research shows that **eating slowly can help us eat less and control weight**. For example, chewing our food twice as long as we normally do helps us control our portion sizes because eating takes longer, which naturally decreases calories consumption.

It takes time (generally about 20–30 minutes) for our brain to signal to our stomach that we are full, which may explain why we feel fuller sooner when we eat more slowly. We end up consuming about ten percent fewer calories when we eat at a slower pace, and presumably chew slower, as opposed to when we rush. After we finish what is on our plate, take a few minutes to drink some water. This simple habit will allow our brain some time to signal our stomach if it's satisfied.

Smart Snacking

The MMD includes two light snacks throughout the day —one at mid morning and the other in the afternoon. In Italian, these are called the *merenda,* and are generally consumed after school by students. A healthy snack would preferably include a yogurt, a piece of fruit, or a few unsalted nuts (about 7–8 walnuts, almonds, hazelnuts, or pistachios, or a handful of pine nuts). This keeps our hormone peaks stable throughout the day, preventing insulin peaks that can lead to weight gain, and it also keeps our appetite under control.

CHAPTER 11

The Benefits of a Home-Cooked Meal

HOW MANY MEALS ARE you eating out per week? If your answer is "three or more meals a week," this is no longer an occasional treat—it is a bad habit!

In the past forty years, we have seen an upward trend in eating out at restaurants. It's understandable; modern life is hectic. Families often have long commutes to work and school, there are often two working parents, and children do plenty of activities after school. The presence of convenient meal options and affordable restaurants is attractive and welcome, we think—but the truth is, it comes at the expense of our health. Fast food, burgers packed with calories but lacking nutritious micronutrients and fiber; pre-packaged frozen meals; dishes from the deli which are heated up in the microwave; even a simple meal at a restaurant, which risks being unnecessarily rich in calories—people are eating out more and cooking less, and the result is perhaps the greatest contributor to lifestyle-related diseases.

Even putting aside the obvious health benefits, learning to cook is a highly useful skill—providing survival knowledge, independence, longevity, and a lot fun, too! If we are always being cooked for, then we won't ever learn these skills and we won't learn new

131

dishes or have the pride of being able to say, "I made this myself." The questions of convenience and home cooking should not be as strongly linked as they are today. Home cooking is should be seen for what it is: an action of love towards ourselves and the people we care about. For many people, cooking is a love-hate relationship, but this dynamic can absolutely be changed. I learned how to cook from my mother and grandmother, and I am now doing the same with my children. This is the way we Italians learn to cook—from generation to generation.

That said, let me reassure you by saying that Italian cuisine is varied yet simple, so with only few ingredients and a little bit of time, you can cook a tasty and healthy meal (which could also be brought to work in a lunch box); you just need a bit of will and creativity! I have provided some examples in this book in Part III: Recipes and Seasonal Menus. I hope my recipes inspire people to cook meals and enjoy the process of cooking from scratch. Take time to prepare your own dishes instead of relying of what the food industry offers. Your health and your wallet will thank you!

Here are my five reasons why preparing food at home is better, and better for you.

Healthier Ingredients and Cooking Techniques

Eating home-cooked food allows us to control not only the ingredients (preferring those which are healthy and high quality), but also the cooking techniques. Food prepared in restaurants or available pre-made at the grocery store is usually high in sodium, "bad" fats (such as saturated fats) or *trans* fats (because they are cheaper), and is rich in sugar and preservatives. It's also possible that the ingredients have been frozen or dried out to provide for a longer shelf life, or the meal could have been prepared days before. Take, for example, an omelet or scrambled eggs. At home, fresh eggs are cracked and other ingredients are added, such as fresh milk, herbs, salt, pepper, and good butter (or extra virgin olive oil) to make a quick and healthy meal. In a café, such a meal could be prepared hours before being cooked, not stored in a refrigerator, cooked using cheap oils, or prepared with excessive salt and substitutes like powdered milk. Eating at home is therefore one of the best ways to promote a healthy lifestyle.

Appropriate Portion Size

When we prepare our food, we are the "boss" of our plate. When we eat out, we have to rely on someone else's choice. The MMD is an inclusive diet, but one key to its success is **MODERATION**. It permits occasional treats, like a glass of wine, and promotes **portion control.** The best way to control our portion size is to use smaller plates, so that the amount of food seems larger (because of an optical illusion called the *Delboeuf Illusion*). So if we put a small amount of pasta, for example, on a large plate, our brain will tell us to put more pasta on the plate. Instead, if we instead put the same amount of pasta on a smaller plate, our mind will tell us that we are eating enough pasta, so we will stop adding more to our plate. We are typically in the habit of "filling" our plate. This is fine: in American and British cuisine, a meal usually comes on one plate, complete with salad, veggies, meat, and carbohydrates. But in Italian cuisine, we tend to serve the parts of the meal separately, on smaller plates, as courses. So using a large plate for meals such as pasta can quickly turn into overeating. This is a simple habit, but it really works! Try it!

In the last fifty years, the food industry has encouraged us to eat more, also increasing the size of plates. Let me give you a simple example. I own a set of china that previously belonged to my grandmother. At first glance, it might seem like an ordinary set of china, but if you look closely, you will notice that the size of the plates is smaller than modern day china plates. In the past, people simply ate less than today and large china was unnecessary.

Removal of Temptations

If we are going on a diet, eating at home can help us stay faithful to our diet program. But when we are eating out, we are exposed to greater temptations—tastier but more unhealthy foods. Also, it is more likely that we "forget" about our dietary restrictions and throw good habits out the window "just this once." The best way to overcome these temptations is to create a lifestyle where it is easy to stay away from them.

Cost Advantages

Another important benefit of eating at home is that we can save money. Pasta, fruits, vegetables, legumes, fish, meat, and other ingredients from grocery stores and local markets are often affordable, and the total cost of a homemade meal is always less than the cost of a meal at a restaurant. This is because a restaurant is designed primarily as a profit-making venture. The owner opened the restaurant to make money, not just for his passion of cooking for others.

Encourages Family Bonding

Eating at home offers an excellent opportunity for family bonding. We can talk to our children about school, or to our partner about our day at work. Dinner in particular is a good time of the day to spend time with your family. There are many reasons for this, which we'll cover a little later in this chapter.

Builds Healthy Habits

Above all, the MMD guidelines should teach you how to create good life-long habits. Diets are usually short-lived and have the opposite effect when the dieter falls back into bad habits. Instead, the MMD is a lifestyle which is easy to adopt. By learning how to cook and eat at home, health and weight take care of themselves, and the skills you learn integrate into your routine for life. By discovering healthy recipes, learning about food and cooking, and creating meal plans, you can be inspired to lead a healthier life.

EAT WHAT YOU LOVE WITH THOSE YOU LOVE

Food is one pleasure of life which embraces all the senses: vision, smell, taste, touch, and hearing. In Italy, we say, "*A tavola non si invecchia*," "One does not grow old at the table." The pleasure of good food, wine and company is such that the passage of time is suspended.

Italian food is not only nourishing, healthy and pleasurable. It also embodies the Italian culture. Just as important as the food's ingredients are the people who prepared it and those who eat it together. Italian food is **FAMILY—conviviality**! This ritual of sharing a meal is a means of bonding and strengthening relationships. During mealtime, we talk and we transmit values, stories, and traditions from generation to generation. I grew up in a family where we ate together as a family for both lunch and dinner, and again for Sunday lunch with relatives and friends. Enjoying our company together was the main ingredient of our meal. I have tried to stick to this routine with my husband and children, especially for dinner and on the weekends when everybody is at home. We sit at the table, enjoy our food, and share our daily lives.

Conviviality is the fulcrum of many social, linguistic, and cultural aspects of Italian life. In fact, UNESCO has defined the Mediterranean diet as: "Eating together is the foundation of the cultural identity and continuity of communities throughout the Mediterranean basin. It is a moment of social exchange and communication."

Several studies have shown that eating together has multiple benefits for everyone involved. There is clear evidence that family meals and shared meals (among adults) are associated with better dietary intake, weight management, and lifestyle.[1] There is another interesting study from the University of Minnesota that looked at family eating habits of nearly 5,000 middle-school students and teenagers, and found that 30 percent ate family meals seven days a week, 30 percent ate family meals twice a week, and the rest never did. The research showed that those who regularly had meals with their parents ate more fruits, vegetables, and calcium-rich foods, ingested more vitamins and nutrients, and consumed less junk food. Some of the research even showed that kids who regularly sit down to a family meal were at lower risk for behaviors like smoking and drug and alcohol use.

Finding the Time

In today's family life, it is not always easy to find the time between work, appointments, homework assignments, and other responsibilities for family to come together at the dinner table to share mealtimes. Yet the ritual of preparing, sharing, and making conversation at the dinner table remains a beneficial option for physical, psychological, and emotional health. What it takes is organization— managing the shopping, preparation, decision of menu, and the final clean-up—but sharing some or all of these tasks brings the family together with an appreciation of the effort, the taste, and the conversation that goes into making a successful family meal.

For those living alone, trying to find someone to eat with isn't always easy. Try to schedule at least some of your mealtimes with family and friends, eating at their home or yours (which can help you hone your own entertaining skills). Another option could be joining a class or volunteering, which can lead to new dining friends.

---

1   Jayne et al., 2014

Above all, try to maintain the habit of eating at the table, whether you are eating alone or with others, rather than on a couch watching TV. It is always better for the digestion and is simply a good habit of etiquette.

Regardless of how you manage it, make the effort to share mealtimes with family or friends. It will demonstrate the true benefits of Italian-style conviviality!

MAKING SMART CHOICES WHEN EATING OUT

Eating out can be a fantastic experience for the palate, providing us with opportunities to try new dishes that would be difficult to make in an everyday kitchen. But despite the opportunities that eating out affords us, it is not always great for our diet or our health. There are many calories and processed ingredients hidden in the cream sauces, cheese fillings, and salad dressings that restaurants use to give their food that rich, memorable taste. Going out once in a while should be seen as a treat—one which we shouldn't deny ourselves, but which should be "on occasion," rather than often. And when it comes to business, in Italy we say, *"I migliori affari si fanno a tavola"*—you do the best business after a good meal, especially with a good wine!

TRATTORIE

A lot of people ask me which restaurants in town are my favorite, which can be difficult to answer when you are used to the taste of home-cooked food. In any case, when I go out with friends I like to find a place where I can eat well and still wake up the next day hungry for a good breakfast. In this pursuit, I find it easier if I avoid chains and instead visit small restaurant like *trattorie*.

A *trattoria* is a family business where a member of the family, usually the *mamma* or *nonna*, cooks in the kitchen while the rest of the family does the managing. It is less formal than a restaurant; the menus are kept small and are normally hand printed, the service is personal and casual, the prices are low, and the food, for the most part, is local and authentic. They prepare fresh food with ingredients available at the local market or from their own garden. Sometimes you can also take the food home; the name *"trattoria"* comes from French *"traiteur,"* meaning a caterer that only makes take-out food.

While you may not have *trattoria* where you live, if you look around, you're almost certain to find small, family-owned restaurants that can offer you the next best thing to a home-cooked meal!

Here are some simple rules to adopt before and at the restaurant to make your meal a pleasant and healthy experience.

Plan ahead. What should you do before going to the restaurant?

Look up the restaurant's menu online to review the options available and make reservations. Waiting at the bar for a table will increase your hunger and you carry the temptation to have an *aperitivo* drink before your meal, often with unhealthy snacks.

Choose starters with caution.

Although they are delicious, these will increase the total amount of calories for your meal. To stay on something healthy, choose vegetables with vinaigrette (in Italy, it this is called *pinzimonio*). They are often accompanied by cold cuts and cheese spreads, but try to stick to vegetables. If there is some cheese in the dish, ask for something light; for example, *feta*.

Choose something healthy.

A large salad is a good choice. Feel free to add some grilled chicken, tuna steak, or good grains (quinoa, spelt, millet, buckwheat). These types of salads are usually my favorite choices. Be careful to order the right sauce and ask for it on the side so that you can add just the right amount. In most restaurants in Italy, salad dressings such as extra virgin olive oil, vinegar, and salt are brought to the table, allowing you to choose your dressing. Avoid fatty salads. This this is a light course, to be kept tasty but healthy. That means avoiding anything in a creamy sauce (like coleslaw, pasta salads, and potato salads). Instead, load up on the raw vegetables, or treat yourself to a few well-drained marinated vegetables (artichoke hearts, red peppers, or mushrooms) and, for a change, add in some fruits or nuts. Also watch out for any the add-ons to vegetable salads. Many salads are come loaded with cheese and cured meat. You can add to your salad some grilled chicken, tuna steak, or good grains.

Choose a simple pasta dish.

If you are craving pasta, choose a very simple one. In any case, I would recommend eating pasta in a restaurant in rather than outside Italy—unless, of course, it is run by Italians. Cooking pasta is an art, and not many restaurants have perfected the skill. Beware of pasta that is overcooked and loaded with sauces, such as Fettucine with Alfredo sauce, spaghetti with meatballs, and macaroni and cheese. However, I would categorize them as more Italian-American; they are not typical of *classic* Italian food. In any case, avoid pasta sauces that contain cream and a lot of fat. It is preferable to choose pasta with tomato sauce or vegetable sauce prepared from scratch. I would also avoid "*Carbonara*" and those sauces made with butter, Parmesan cheese, and cream. If you're concerned about the amount of carbs you are having, it is better you stick to grilled meat, fish, and vegetables.

Go for chicken, fish or beef.

Ask for grilled, not fried or stir-fried. Avoid the breading and the fillings. As a side dish, remain faithful to salads or vegetables instead of French fries or potatoes *au gratin* with cheese.

What about pizza?

If it is the pizza day, choose a good "*pizzeria*," or a place where they specialize in pizza, and then order the simplest one: usually "*pizza Napol,*", with which comes with tomato, oregano, garlic (optional), and anchovies without mozzarella cheese; a lot of taste for an adequate number of calories. If you cannot resist the fancier ones, ask for a small pizza with simple toppings like tomato sauce, mozzarella, oregano, and basil, or grilled vegetables, like "*pizza margherita*" or *pizza with vegetables.*

Be smart and play with portions.

Consider splitting a meal or ask to take home half your meal home if you think it's too much to eat in one sitting. Be mindful, take your time, and focus on the company and conversation, not just the food. Stop eating when you are just starting to feel mildly full. Drink water between bites; it will help to fill you up and slow you down. Also, go easy on the booze.

Skip fancy drinks and soft drinks.

If you want to order an alcoholic drink, forget the margaritas, pina colas, and other exotic mixed drinks. They include sugary additions that only add calories. Opt instead for a glass of good wine, a light beer, or a simple Martini or Aperol Spritz (if you crave an *aperitivo*).

Skip a rich dessert.

You can always have some sorbet or some fresh fruit to cap off your meal, much better health-wise than the triple chocolate cake or a mountain of ice cream topped with whipped cream. If you are really craving cake, split it with someone.

Absolutely skip a cappuccino after your meal.

Cappuccino is a morning treat that you should not drink after a meal because it is not good for the digestion (it's too rich). Instead, order an espresso or regular coffee, which helps digestion.

CHAPTER 12

The Basics of Healthy Sleep

I T IS GENERALLY ACCEPTED that in order to live a healthy life, we have to eat well and exercise regularly. However, **sufficient sleep** is just as important for overall health.

The way we think about sleep has changed over time. Many people think of sleep like a necessary evil—time that we are obliged to waste every night. We sleep a lot less than people did hundreds of years ago, which owes a lot to the invention of the electric light. Thanks to easy, plentiful lighting, we are able to be much more productive at later and earlier hours of the day. We can now wake up earlier for work, work longer hours, and stay up later, which is particularly beneficial during winter months. In fact, it has become expected of us to rise before the sun and stay awake for hours after it has gone down.

But this productivity comes at a cost to our health.

On average, we need eight hours of sleep every day, though that amount changes from person to person. Some people need about nine hours of sleep per night to function properly; other people, only six or seven. Getting to sleep at the same time each night helps the heart recover from the day and reduces the risk of heart disease. If you enjoy working out, bear in mind that your muscles only start to repair themselves once you have fallen asleep, preparing you to do the same thing again tomorrow. The regeneration period of the body goes from about 10 pm to 6 am, depending on the individual and the season. Don't panic if once in a while you have a late night; having fun and enjoying life is also part of a healthy Italian lifestyle. But the greatest message you can take from the MMD guide is to build good overall health habits.

WHY IS SLEEP SO IMPORTANT?

The reason sleep is so important is because it is the time when our body is able to grow, repair itself, and heal. Getting enough quality sleep at the right times can help protect our physical health, mental health, and overall quality of life.

Nearly all living things follow circadian rhythms, or a "body clock," which synchronizes bodily functions to the 24-hour pattern of the Earth's rotation. In humans, this clock is regulated by the body's senses: most importantly, by the way the eye perceives light and dark and the way our skin feels temperature changes. If we do not sleep a certain amount each night, we are essentially tricking our body into having an unstable circadian rhythm, which can have a lot of health consequences.

Increased Risk of Obesity

The hormones that regulate appetite and inhibit hunger are produced while our body sleeps. There are two main hormones which help us balance energy: ghrelin and leptin. **Ghrelin**, the hunger hormone, is a peptide produced in the stomach that regulates appetite and body weight. When the stomach is empty, ghrelin is secreted, which signals the brain to understand that we are hungry. When the stomach is stretched, ghrelin secretion stops. It acts on hypothalamic brain cells to increase hunger and increase gastric acid secretion, as well as gastrointestinal motility, to prepare the body for food intake.

Leptin is a hormone which acts in the contrary to ghrelin: it signals satiety, or fullness. It is a peptide released by fatty tissue and regulates energy balance by inhibiting hunger. Obese individuals tend to experience a decreased sensitivity to leptin, resulting in an inability to detect satiety after eating despite high energy stores. During sleep, the levels of ghrelin decrease, because sleep requires less energy than being awake, so it isn't necessary to signal hunger. People who don't sleep enough have less of these low-ghrelin hours, and so end up with too much ghrelin. As a result, the body thinks it is hungry and in need of more energy, so it stops burning calories because it thinks there is a shortage. A recent prospective study reported that shorter sleep duration was associated with a 45 percent increased risk of obesity.[1]

Stress Hormone Levels are Increased

Upregulated stress hormones are associated with insulin resistance, which leads to type 2 diabetes. It is also associated with weight gain and obesity, which are linked to many other lifestyle related conditions.

Immune System Function is Suppressed

The more all-nighters we pull, the more likely we are to decrease our body's ability to respond to bacterial and viral infections, meaning we'll easily suffer from every cold and flu that comes our way. When we sleep, we actively fight off foreign pathogens. But by burning the candle at both ends, we give ourselves less recovery time and end up fighting pathogens passively while we are awake, which is much less efficient.

---

1 Wu et Zhai, 2014

Muscle Recovery After Physical Exercise is Prevented

Whether our goal in the gym is losing weight, building muscle, becoming more flexible, running a faster time, or simply warding off poor health, all physical activity requires us to use our muscles. Imagine your muscles as networks of fibers which, upon exercise, are pulled apart here and there. The more strenuous the activity, the more these fibers are broken apart. When we sleep, these fibers are able to knit themselves back together thanks to the extra energy made available by resting. Amino acids, the building blocks of protein, are the raw materials which muscle is made from. By consuming protein-rich meals, particularly before bed time, we have sufficient material to work with overnight to repair muscle tears. In addition, while we sleep, we are signaling our body hormonally to increase protein synthesis pathways, which means we create more protein from amino acids for building and repairing tissue such as muscle. We also decrease protein degradation pathways, which recycle muscle. Sufficient sleep and adequate protein intake helps avoid the loss of muscle mass and aids with muscle recovery caused by exercise, injury, or health conditions. So, with a good night's sleep and a decent dinner, our physical activity goals can be met.

Human Growth Hormone Levels are Negatively Impacted

Human growth hormone (GH) is another hormone which is released under conditions of sleep. In men, sixty to seventy percent of daily human GH secretion occurs during the early hours of sleep, which is typically when the deepest sleep cycles occur.

TIPS FOR POOR SLEEPERS

Falling asleep can seem an impossible dream when you are lying awake at 2 AM, but you can experiment with some of the following tips, to find the ones that work for you:

 Get as much **natural light and fresh air** as possible each day.

 Get plenty of **physical exercise every day.** Ensure you time exercise properly. It is better to exercise in the morning or early in the afternoon, as strenuous exercise too close to bed can interfere with sleep.

3 **Limit caffeine, alcohol, smoking, and the consumption of a heavy dinner, snacks,** and **sugar** before bedtime.

4 Make sure your **bedroom is quiet and dark.**

5 **Avoid excessive fluid** intake in the evening, such as water and herbal tea. Drinking too much just before going to bed may result in several trips to the bathroom throughout the night. I often drink a relaxing herbal tea containing chamomile, lemon balm, linden, and fennel 1½ hours before going to bed. In the same way that a cappuccino is my morning pleasure, herbal tea is my evening pleasure!

6 **Clear your head.** Stress, anxiety, and anger accumulated during the day may make it difficult to fall asleep. Try to relax yourself by listening to classic music or reading a book. Personally, after only 15 minutes of reading I fall fast asleep—*buona notte!*

CHAPTER 13

Tips for Increasing Metabolism

O UR BASAL METABOLIC RATE (BMR) is the minimum amount of energy required to maintain the vital functions in our body, both at complete rest and when fasting. These vital processes include keeping our heart beating, breathing, blood flowing, cell growth, brain and nerve functioning, and muscle movement. It's the energy you would use if you were just lying in bed all day; going running, walking to work, or even sitting in your office chair, which would burn a little more, isn't included. BMR affects the rate at which we burn calories and whether we maintain, gain, or lose weight. Our BMR accounts for about 60–75 percent of the calories we burn every day, depending on whether and how much we exercise. BMR is directly correlated to body surface and increases with body weight and dimension; interestingly, an overweight or obese person has a higher BMR than a lean person because they have more tissue requiring circulation and more weight to move when they perform simple actions.

There are **several factors that can influence BMR**:

1. **Age.** BMR is highest during periods of rapid growth. As we get older, unfortunately, the amount of muscle decreases and metabolism naturally slows by about 2–5 percent per decade after age 40 due to a decrease in lean mass. To better maintain BMR, physical activity is highly recommended for the elderly.

2. **Gender.** Males generally have a higher BMR than females.

3. **Climate.** BMR increases in cold climates.

4. **Body mass.** BMR is higher in muscular people, and, to a lesser degree, in overweight people.

5. **Hormones.** The thyroid hormones **triiodothyronine (T3)** and **thyroxine (T4)** are the principal regulators of metabolic rate. When the supply of thyroid hormones is inadequate, BMR may fall by between 30–50 percent. If the thyroid is hyperactive, BMR may increase to twice the normal value.

6. **Pregnancy.** BMR increases during pregnancy, especially in the final stages of gestation, and then even more during breastfeeding.

7. **Starvation.** If our body perceives starvation, either by real or by extreme dieting, BMR can drop by as much as 50 percent below normal. Diets below 1,000 calories a day can decrease metabolic rate. The body is programmed for survival and interprets the reduction in calories as starvation, and all systems slow down to conserve energy. This is the reason why simple calorie restriction is an insufficient method to use for weight loss, and instead it is **always important to follow a balanced diet that provides the right nutrients and the right number of calories according to our BMR**. In average-size male and female adults, the energy expended on just BMR is about 1,650 and 1,350 kilocalories a day, respectively. **One of the most effective remedies to lose weight is to increase our BMR.**

There are two major "tricks" that we can adopt to naturally increase our BMR: **eating properly and being physical active**.

EATING PROPERLY

A balanced diet, like the MMD, is the key to naturally improving one's BMR, following the body's physiology. By adjusting our diet and choosing the right foods that will help us speed up our metabolism more easily, we allow ourselves greater control over our weight without too many sacrifices and while still enjoying food.

First of all, we should **distribute the amount of macronutrients** without excluding any of them (carbohydrates, lipids, and protein) throughout the day following the rule of 3 + 2 (three meals + two snacks; you can read more about it on page 303). Each meal should contain **protein**, because protein helps build lean body mass, which increases BMR. This is very important because, unlike carbohydrates and lipids, there is no amino acids storage in our body; therefore, we must consume amino acids for them to be present in the blood in the right quantity during the whole day. Protein percentages at dinner should be a little bit higher than at lunch, because muscle repairs and growth occurs during sleep. Protein quality is also important; this means you should opt for foods like **fish, eggs, lean meat (preferably poultry), and legumes**, which have a great variety and density of essential amino acids.

Besides protein, there are some foods that increase body mass more than others, and therefore can help us reach our goals more easily. It is important to underline the role of omega-3 polyunsaturated fatty acids (PUFAs) and their metabolites in increasing metabolism. These molecules are natural ligands for peroxisome proliferator-activated receptors (PPAR-α). When they are activated, enhancing energetic metabolism, they increase fat-burning capacity. Consequently, a diet with the right percentage of food containing PUFAs, including **oil, fish, beans, soybeans, and nuts**, helps us burn more calories, which is useful to increase metabolism.

Ingredients for Boosting BMR

Many spices have been used for centuries to add taste and flavor to food. Several studies showed that tasty spices are beneficial for burning calories, including **cinnamon, hot chili pepper, and pepper**, which have been used in Mediterranean cuisine for centuries. Ginger and turmeric, which come from Asia, are also present in our cuisine and are useful for increasing burning fat. All of these spices can promote **thermogenesis** (heat production), increase satiety, and contribute to weight loss. I usually buy my spices at the local market and keep them in glass jars to preserve all the nutrients. When purchasing spices, always make sure to check the origin and quality.

Cinnamon

This aromatic and flavorsome spice traces its roots back to Egypt. It was also used by the Romans, not only for culinary purposes, but as a medicine, too. Today it is still used in Italian cuisine and is one of my favorite spices for its lightly sugary taste. Research has shown that cinnamon has **anti-microbial as well as anti-parasitic properties**. It also contains **antioxidants, can aid in wound healing, and may even lower blood pressure and LDL-cholesterol**.[1] Cinnamon can help assist in your efforts to **maintain a healthy body weight**. In fact, cinnamon has the unique ability to imitate the activity of insulin in the body, maintaining a regulated blood sugar level.[2] The consumption of cinnamon also speeds our metabolism up (500 mg to 6 g per day for a duration lasting from 40 days to 4 months).[3] It can even slow down the process of moving food into your stomach. This is a good thing if you are attempting to lose weight, because this will help you feel fuller for a longer period of time. In addition, the

---

1   Rahman et al., 2013
2   Pallavi and Rathai, 2015
3   Medagama, 2015

sweet nature of cinnamon can help alleviate a sweet craving. When you are on a weight loss diet, sweets are often off-limits, so cinnamon can fill this void so that we do not feel tempted to reach for high-calorie desserts.

Hot Chili Pepper

Capsaicin is the compound found in hot chili peppers which burns our mouth when we eat it. Not everyone likes it, but I certainly do! In controlled doses, the mouth feel of capsaicin can be pleasant for some. Capsaicin has been shown to **slow down aging** in two ways: it supposedly contains **"longevity molecules"** which could make you live longer by promoting vascular health, and it mimics the effects of caloric restriction. Capsaicin increases the activity of AMPK protein (AMP-activated protein kinase, which plays a key role as a master regulator of cellular energy homeostasis), decreasing the expression of certain gerontogenes implicated in aging. In addition to prolonging life, capsaicin also **reduces appetite**. An intake of 1 mg of hot chili pepper after a meal seems to reduce the levels of ghrelin (the hormone involved in body weight control) and increase satiety.

Capsaicin also acts on **cholesterol and triglycerides**, with no effect on HDL, our "good" cholesterol. Several studies have shown that a diet based on hot chili pepper may prevent atherosclerosis, or plaque in the arteries, that is formed by the oxidation of the LDL-proteins. Hot chili pepper is a very versatile spice to use in the kitchen: it can be enjoyed fresh, dried, cooked, or raw, to flavor and spice up meat, fish, pasta, or sauces. In Italy it is widely used in Calabria—for example, for the typical 'nduja (a typical Calabrese spicy salame)—and throughout the south of Italy, where they love spicy food. It gives such a unique flavor to recipes that when you start using it, you'll never go back.

Black Pepper

Black pepper (*Piper nigrum*) is a flowering vine cultivated for its fruit, which is usually dried and used as a spice and seasoning. Peppercorns, and the ground pepper derived from them, may be described simply as pepper, or more precisely as black pepper (when prepared using cooked and dried unripe fruit), green pepper (using dried unripe fruit) and white pepper (taken from ripe fruit seeds). Pepper increases the hydrochloric acid secretion in the stomach, thereby **facilitating digestion**. Pepper **can also prevent and repair the damage caused by free radicals**. A remarkable reduction in triglycerides and LDL-cholesterol in blood plasma, and better lipid profiles of people treated with black pepper, has been demonstrated. Piperine, present in dietary black pepper, has fat reducing and lipid-lowering effects at a small dose of 40 mg/kg. It has also been shown to have significant **anti-obesity activity**.[4] The piperine molecule found in various forms of pepper enhances the bioavailability of a number of drugs, including curcumin present in turmeric, which increases its bioavailability by twenty-fold.[5]

Ginger

Ginger is the rhizome, or stem, of the *Zingiber officinale* plant, which belongs primarily to Asian traditions where it has been used for centuries as a food, spice and medicine. Recently, it has been introduced into Italian cuisine for its delicious taste and health benefits. Ginger has **digestive, antioxidant, anti-inflammatory,** and **thermogenic properties**, and **promotes feelings of satiety**. Claims that ginger may increase metabolism rates by 20 percent are based on animal studies where a concentrated ginger extract was applied to external tissues. However, consumed internally, even in high doses, ginger

---

4 Shah et al., 2011
5 Patil et al., 2016

does not appear to increase metabolism beyond 2 percent. Of course, any increase in metabolism can help us to stay healthy, especially if combined with a balanced diet and sufficient physical activity.

We can consume ginger in a variety of ways, especially freshly-ground in recipes such as salads, fish, and poultry. I also like to add freshly sliced raw ginger to my lemon and mint tea; others use it in black tea. It is good to flavor water with in the summer, as it is very refreshing. But in order **to better increase metabolism and burn fat, ginger is often combined with garlic, cayenne pepper, cinnamon, turmeric, or green tea** for synergistic effects, as all these ingredients have thermogenic properties.

Turmeric

Turmeric has been used for over 4,000 years to treat many diseases in Chinese medicine and widely grows in different part of Asia and Africa. Turmeric comes from the underground stem of the *Curcuma longa* plant, which is in the ginger family. It can be purchased as a root or, more commonly, as a powder. This bright yellow spice may help our body burn fat. In fact, **curcumin**—the active ingredient in turmeric—increases body heat, which in turn can boost metabolism. The spice also has a host of other health benefits, from **helping fight Alzheimer's disease and infections to reducing inflammation and treating digestive problems.**[6] Try to add turmeric to soups, stews, or roasted chicken, or sprinkle some over roasted veggies or nuts, and the taste of your dishes will turn colorfully delicious.

In addition to healthful spices, some other ingredients to add to your plate to boost BMR include:

Adding nuts to your plate. Contrary to what you might think, **nuts** (in particular almonds, pistachios, walnuts, and pine nuts) are a great source of "good" fats and can help maintain a healthy body

6 Aggarwal 2010; Pulido-Moran et al., 2016

weight. Oils derived from nuts are able to create a **perfect balance between omega-6 and omega-3 FAs** in our body. Obviously, like any other food, don't exaggerate the quantity because they are caloric in nature.

Enjoy seeds in your salad. Seeds are another excellent choice for speeding up metabolism. Sesame, flax, sunflower, and pumpkin seeds are rich in heart-healthy fats that keep us feeling satisfied and energized.

Drink green tea. Green tea is rich in antioxidants, increases thermogenesis, and aids fatty acid degradation. The effect is mediated by two main components: **caffeine and catechin,** which are associated with **energy expenditure**.[7]

PHYSICAL ACTIVITY FOR BOOSTING METABOLISM

Remember that BMR is a measure of only the energy required to keep us alive. So, when we calculate our energy needs, we need to consider all physical activity on top of this; even sitting quietly in a chair burns slightly above one's BMR. A sedentary person usually requires about 30 percent more calories above their BMR to meet their energy needs, whereas a moderately active person might need 40–50 percent more, an active person 75 percent, and a very active person may need double. For example, according to the Italian LARN (Nutritional Society), a sedentary male adult needs about 1800–2000 calories a day, while a female adult about 1600–1800 calories a day. Those participating in high-intensity exercise every day, such as weight lifters or rowers, may consume as many as 4000 calories a day! The most effective way to "boost" our metabolism is to participate in both cardio training and resistance training, which together provide a protective effect against a drop in metabolism.

---

7 Türközü and Tek, 2017

This is because people tend to lose a considerable portion of muscle as they age and in calorie-reduction programs that don't include strength training, whereas one of the main benefits from exercise is the preservation of muscle.

Eating well, together with physical activity, is the key to making the Mamma Mia Diet successful; one without the other it is nowhere near as effective. When it comes to weight control, research has indicated that diet accounts for 60–70 percent of progress, while physical activity is responsible for the remaining 30–40 percent (although this statistic varies between individuals).

Regular exercise is important for our physical fitness and our general health. It can help prevent and manage a range of health problems, it improves mood, and it boosts our energy levels. We Italians walk, ride our bikes, and take the stairs much more often than other cultures, who instead use cars and escalators. Part of the reason for this is that many Italians live in pedestrian cities, which have been built for walking and cycling; in fact, many city centers that were previously adapted for automobile use are now being closed to vehicular traffic and are being returned to the pedestrians! It is also common to see Italians taking a walk in the afternoon or after dinner, especially in summer and on the weekends, with their family and friends—the so-called "*Passeggiata in centro*," an enjoyable addition to regular daily physical activity.

In contrast to this, recent research on more than one million adults found that sitting for more than eight hours a day increases the risk of premature death by up to 60 percent. In fact, physical inactivity has been identified as the fourth leading risk factor for global mortality after high blood pressure, tobacco use, and high blood glucose.

The World Health Organization recommends at least **thirty minutes of moderate-intensity physical activity** five times a week to keep us in good health, and **forty-five minutes of intense exercise** three times a week. **It is very important to plan time for this level of activity and include it in our weekly schedule as part of** our lifestyle. **As a result of following these guidelines, we will be in good shape, live longer and be happier.** And remember: these guidelines are for the minimum amount for good health; those who take the initiative to integrate more physical activity into their lives certainly stand to benefit more and can even free themselves from some health concerns for life.

The Difference between Physical Activity and Exercise

Physical activity is defined as movement that involves contractions of our muscles. Many activities we do regularly every day involve movement, such as housework, walking to work, climbing stairs, and gardening. On the other hand, **exercise** is a planned physical activity, performed intentionally with a fitness-related goal, such as working out, swimming, cycling, running, or playing tennis or golf. It's necessary to get both types of activity, no matter what stage of life you're at.

Here are 10 important reasons to be physically active:

1 It keeps you healthier and reduces the risk of many health conditions; for example, cardiovascular disease, obesity, type 2 diabetes, osteoporosis, and cancer.

2 Increase your chances of living longer.

3 Feel better about yourself. Look good and in shape, which also offers emotional benefits.

4 Reduce your risk of depression.

5 Sleep better at night.

6 Get around better (better mobility).

7 Have stronger muscles and bones. More muscle burns more calories, plus it reduces the risk of developing osteoporosis.

⑧   Achieve and maintain a healthy weight.

⑨   Spend quality time with friends or meet new people.

⑩   Be more in contact with nature through outdoor training.

"Cardio vs Strength Training" Debate

For ages the question has been asked: "Should I focus on cardio training or strength training in my workouts?" The short answer is, "Both."

A fitness plan that includes both cardio and strength training is the most effective. **Cardio training** is any exercise that raises your heart rate and makes your circulatory system stronger by delivering more oxygen to cells. Examples include running/jogging, swimming, cycling, dancing, rowing, and high-intensity walking. Many low- to medium-intensity cardio activities can be performed for hours on end, and can be therapeutic (such as swimming, which is good for the elderly) and can even be used for physiotherapy (such as cycling to rehabilitate the knees).

Resistance (or strength) training--for example, lifting weights at the gym—is the number-one activity to build more muscles and can even, when done properly, act as a form of aerobic exercise. Strength training is any type of exercise that uses resistance to induce muscular contraction, which in turn builds the strength, anaerobic endurance, and size of muscles. This form of exercise also helps prevent osteoporosis and improves your range of motion and ability to perform day-to-day movements.

Scientific research has largely supported the use of resistance training to promote fat loss and weight control, confirming its effectiveness through a vast number of studies. Several U.S. health organizations have even introduced this type of training into their programs for maintaining good health[8]. Resistance training is an

8 Kraemer et al., 2002

essential component of any weight management program due to its important role in maintaining and/or increasing body mass by building muscle, which is much more effective than cardio training alone.[9]

Muscle mass also contributes significantly to increasing a person's BMR, as muscle is active tissue compared to fatty tissue and consequently increases the energy expended to maintain all bodily functions. Resistance training is also able to promote lipid oxidation (fat burning) for up to 24 hours after the activity has stopped, giving this type of training an important role in preventing the accumulation of fat and obesity.[10]

You can now see the benefits of both types of exercise, so know to combine cardio and resistance training for the most effective results. Ask your trainer to prepare an adequate program for you according to your sex, age, and physical conditions which combines both types of training.

9 Hunter et al., 2008
10 Hansen et al., 2005

STICK TO THE PROGRAM

Have you ever failed in keeping up with a new exercise program? For many people, starting is easy, but maintenance is hard part—and the key to success. We have to start slowly and remain motivated, constant, and disciplined.

The worst enemy is time. Watch out for the usual excuses: "I don't have time," "I'm too busy with work, family, etc." Rather than thinking about exercise as lost time, look at it as gained health; physical activity is an opportunity, not an inconvenience. In Italy, it is common to walk or bike to work. This may not be an option available to everyone, but the point of the Italian lifestyle is to integrate exercise and physical activity into your routines so that you can function healthily on autopilot. Viable alternatives might be a brisk thirty-minute walk in the neighborhood before work, or stopping in at the gym on the way to your workplace. This is what I do regularly, and I feel full of energy for the rest of my day!

A Few Exercise Tips

Although moderate physical activity is safe for most people, health experts suggest that you talk to your doctor before committing to any exercise program, especially if any of the following conditions apply to you: heart disease, asthma or lung disease, type 1 or type 2 diabetes, kidney disease, arthritis, or if you are being treated for cancer or have recently completed cancer treatment.

If you're having trouble getting your exercise in, try doing some of the following:

1. Set some easy goals at the beginning; for example, 15 minutes walking at a fast pace every day for one week. Then, increase the duration by 5 minutes each week until you reach at least 30 minutes a day. Aim for 1 hour a day, 3 days a week. Walking burns calories, and the faster you walk, the more you burn. Remember that speed isn't the only factor controlling weight by walking. You have to reach 65–70 percent of your body's maximum heart rate to substantially improve your fitness and burn serious calories.

2. Be realistic when creating a plan. Set achievable goals so you won't be demotivated, and try to stick to your program for a few weeks. Then move to the next goal; your body needs to be "surprised" every once in a while.

3. Try to find a friend to exercise with you. You will motivate each other. If you feel comfortable doing so, join a gym or a sports club.

4. Maintain healthy habits! It is challenging, but they say it takes about two months to make a new habit, so stick it out. Rewarding yourself with something you like for your healthy efforts (though never with food) will reinforce your new habits and inspire you to continue your journey.

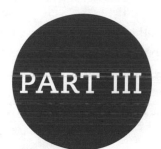

PART III

Recipes and
Seasonal Menus

THE RECIPES IN THIS book are easy to make, and most of them are fast to prepare; no special culinary skills are needed. They are suitable for the modern lifestyle in which people do not have so much time for cooking, as they did in the past. I have chosen them with passion, trying to include many of the regional traditions of Italy, from the north to the south, some of them belonging to my family's own culinary tradition. I have added a "Mamma Mia!" note to each recipe, containing some nutritional, historical, personal, and geographical information to provide information on the ingredients, as well as substitutes that may be more easily found in other countries. These tips will help you have more fun when preparing these Italian dishes in your kitchen, minimizing stress and maximizing enjoyment.

Remember, Italian cuisine, at its heart, requires only three things: "*Pasta, amore e fantasia,*" —pasta, love and creativity, and you are ready to go!

I have divided the recipes into categories like Breakfast, Lunch, and Dinner to help you construct a balanced daily menu. I have also included four sample seasonal daily menus at the end of this section to give you an idea of how to combine tasty and healthy meals during different periods of the year.

BREAKFAST

HOMEMADE LOW SUGAR JAM

Total preparation time: **1 hour and 50 minutes**
Cooking time: **40 minutes**
Yield: **About 16–17 oz (450–480 g)**

Jam jars, sterilized
18 oz (500 g) apricots, nectarines or strawberries, cleaned,
    washed, dried and cut into small pieces
¼ cup (50 g) granulated sugar
1 small organic golden delicious apple, washed, dried and cut
    into small pieces
½ organic medium lemon, juiced
3 tablespoons water

1   In a large bowl, combine the fruits and the lemon juice. Mix
     well and cover with plastic wrap. Let rest at room temperature
     for 1 hour.

2   Pour the fruit in a medium-sized saucepan before adding the
     sugar and the water. Cook on medium-low heat for about
     35–40 minutes, stirring occasionally to prevent the mixture
     from sticking to the bottom of the pan.

3   Remove from heat and let rest for a few minutes. Purée the
     fruit using a food mill or, if possible, a food processor (to
     retain more of the fiber content).

4   Pour the warm fruit jam into hot jars (previously sterilized,
     with new caps) and fill them up, leaving a gap of about ½ inch
     (about 1 cm). Seal and turn upside down for about 10 minutes
     to create a vacuum.

5   Allow them to cool. You can keep fruit jam in the refrigerator
     for several weeks, but once opened, you'll need to use it within
     3–4 days.

MAMMA MIA!

The fruit is the star of this recipe. Once you've got the right, perfectly ripe fruit, you are good to go. Avoid over-ripe fruit, which will lead to overcooked flavors, a leathery texture, and will lack some of the pectin and acidity that are essential for good jams. In fact, the addition of a golden delicious apple to this recipe is due to its **high amount of pectin** (especially in the skin). Pectin is a **naturally occurring polysaccharide with thickening and gelling properties**. Pectin requires both heat and acid (which is why it is important to add lemon juice). My recipe also calls for a small amount of **added sugar**, to sweeten the deal.

HOMEMADE MUESLI

Total preparation time: **10 minutes**
Baking time: **6–8 minutes**
Yield: **25 oz (700 g)**

2 tablespoons coconut oil
½ cup (about 50 g) dried unsweetened coconut flakes
⅓ heaping cup (50 g) sunflower seeds
¼ cup (about 25 g) flax seeds
½ cup (about 60 g) almonds, coarsely chopped
½ cup (about 60 g) hazelnuts, coarsely chopped
1¼ cups (about 135 g) oatmeal
½ heaping cup (about 85 g) raisins
½ heaping cup (about 85 g) dried cranberries
½ cup (about 100 g) dried apricots, coarsely chopped
A pinch of nutmeg (optional)
Fresh fruit, milk or yogurt to serve

1   Preheat the oven to 350°F (180°C). Place some parchment paper on a baking sheet and set the oven rack to middle position.

2   In a small sauce pan, melt coconut oil *without* boiling it.

3   In a bowl, mix sunflower seeds, flax seeds, almonds, and hazelnuts. Drizzle with coconut oil.

4   Mix well and spread out in a thin layer on the baking sheet. Toast for 6–8 minutes, mixing twice, until all nuts are toasted. Remove from oven and let cool completely on a cooling grid.

5   In a large bowl, mix coconut flakes, oatmeal, raisins, cranberries, and apricots. Then, add toasted ingredients and a pinch of nutmeg.

6   Mix well and keep in an airtight container for up to 10–12 days. Serve with fresh fruit (such as pomegranate, strawberries, or blueberries) and milk or yogurt.

MAMMA MIA!

This is an incredibly **nutritious breakfast**, full of **fiber, protein, healthy fats,** and **carbohydrates**. I prefer toasting the seeds and nuts to enhance their flavors, though you can omit this step to save time. Muesli is an uncooked mixture of grains, dried fruits, nuts, and seeds, typical of Germany but also common to the northern part of Italy called *Sud-Tirol*. Muesli can be mixed with milk, yogurt, and fresh squeezed fruit juices, or eaten *al naturale* (no soaking). However, soaking is beneficial because it helps to reduce the amount of **phytic acid**, a compound naturally present in grains, nuts, soybeans, legumes, and seeds. Phytic acid binds to minerals such as zinc iron, phosphorus, calcium, and magnesium, decreasing their absorption rates. The amount of phytic acid in muesli can be highly reduced by soaking, as well as by fermenting, sprouting or cooking. That said, for those who have a **balanced omnivore diet**, the deficiencies caused by phytic acid are **not a concern**. In fact, consumption of certain high-phytate foods as part of a **balanced diet** has numerous benefits.

OATMEAL AND BANANA CAKE

Total preparation time: **20 minutes**
Baking time: **15 minutes**
Yield: **2 servings**

1¼ cups (135 g) oatmeal flakes
¼ heaping cup (about 50 g) dried cranberries or raisins
¼ heaping cup (about 45 g) toasted almonds or toasted
    hazelnuts, coarsely chopped
2 ripe large bananas, mashed
½ large apple, peeled and finely sliced
⅓ cup (80 ml) almond milk
¼–½ teaspoon cinnamon (or to taste)

1   Preheat the oven to 350°F (180°C). Set oven rack to middle
    position.

2   In a medium bowl, mix together oatmeal, cranberries,
    almonds, and cinnamon.

3   Add milk and mix well (the amount of milk may vary depend-
    ing on the type of the oatmeal flakes).

4   Let the mixture rest for a few minutes, allowing the oatmeal
    to soak up the milk (it should be wet), then add bananas
    and apple. Pour into a 5 x 7 in. (13 x 18 cm) oiled or nonstick
    baking pan.

5   Bake for about 10–15 minutes, until lightly brown on top. Cut
    into squares and serve either warm or at room temperature.
    You can store for up to 1–2 days in the refrigerator.

MAMMA MIA!

Oatmeal—tasty, healthy and quick—is loaded in dietary fiber (in particular beta-glucan, which is known to **help lower LDL cholesterol**—the bad cholesterol). Not only that, oatmeal is rich in protein, minerals (in particular, manganese, selenium, phosphorus, and zinc), vitamins (in particular, carotenoids, vitamin E, and flavonoids) and is low in fat. Fiber helps keep you satiated so you are less likely to overeat; in fact, simply adding more fiber to your diet is one of the easiest ways to shed pounds. Oatmeal also has a relatively **low Glycemic Index (GI)**; therefore, it is suitable for diabetics. Oatmeal plays an important role in managing **metabolic syndrome.**

Bananas, another key element of this dish, are one of the most widely consumed fruits in the world—and for good reason. Bananas are **rich in potassium,** which can lower blood pressure. Unripe bananas contain more starch than some other fruits (70–80 percent); however, during ripening, the starch is converted into sugar and ends up being less than 1 percent when the banana is fully ripe. Bananas have a **Glycemic Index (GI) of 42–70**, depending on their ripeness (an unripe banana would be 42 and a ripe banana, 70). Bananas are also a good source of other types of fiber, such as pectin. Both **pectin and resistant starch moderate blood sugar levels after meals.**

PEACH SHAKE

Preparation time: **5 minutes**
Yield: **2 servings**

3 peeled medium peaches or 3 unpeeled medium nectarines,
    sliced
1 medium banana, sliced
2 large dates, pitted and coarsely chopped
1 cup (240 ml) almond milk
¼ teaspoon vanilla extract
1 pinch of cinnamon (optional)

1   Cut all fruits in pieces.

2   Place all ingredients in a blender and blend until smooth. You
     might need to add 1–2 extra tablespoons of milk, depending
     on the size of the fruits. Serve immediately.

MAMMA MIA!

Peaches are typical summer fruits in Italy. Juicy and rich in water, they are perfect for a summer diet! Peaches are **highly satiating, with a low GI (42)** to help keep hunger at bay for longer periods, making them a good choice to incorporate into a **weight loss die**t.

The addition of **almond milk** adds delicious flavor to this shake and makes it suitable for a **lactose-free diet**. The almond taste blends well with the sweet flavor and fragrant aroma of peaches. You can substitute almond milk with cow's milk if you are not lactose intolerant.

Dates originated around the Nile and Euphrates rivers of ancient Egypt and Mesopotamia. Now, however, the date palm grows in warm climates on all continents. Wonderfully delicious, dates are one the most popular fruits in the world, packing a ton of **fiber, vitamins** (pro-vitamin A), **antioxidants,** and **minerals.** An excellent source of **iron**, dates also contain calcium, phosphorus, potassium, and zinc. I love dates, whether by themselves, stuffed, in sweets, or in shakes like this one!

POACHED EGG, MASHED AVOCADO, AND TOAST

Total preparation time: **10 minutes**
Cooking time: **3–4 minutes**
Yield: **2 servings**

2 slices whole grain bread
2 large very fresh eggs
1 tablespoon white vinegar
2 medium ripe Roma tomatoes, peeled and diced into small
    pieces
¼ medium red onion, coarsely grated
¼ ripe avocado
½ organic lime, juice
Extra virgin olive oil
Freshly ground pepper, to taste

1   In a bowl, mix tomatoes, onion, a little bit of olive oil (about 1
    teaspoon) and ½ the lime juice. Add some pepper to taste.

2   Fill a wide pan with water. Add vinegar and bring to simmer
    over medium heat. Turn down to low and let the water come
    to a brisk simmer. Using a slotted spoon, create a reel.

3   Crack one of the eggs into a cup. Gently pour the egg into the
    water in one fluid movement. Cook for about 3–4 minutes.
    Remove with a slotted spoon and let it rest on paper towels for
    a few minutes. Repeat with the other egg.

4   Peel, destone, and mash avocado with remaining lime juice.

5   Toast bread.

6   Heat eggs in boiling water for 15 seconds.

7   Spread ½ mashed avocado on each slice of bread before add-
    ing tomatoes and onion. Unwrap your eggs and place on top.

MAMMA MIA!

Avocado makes for a healthy choice; avocados are a great source of several **vitamins, minerals** and **good fats,** in addition to being low in carbs and a **great source of fiber.** Unlike most other fruits, however, avocado is relatively high in fat: mostly monounsaturated fat, plus a small amount of saturated fat and polyunsaturated fat. Several studies have also shown that replacing some saturated fat in one's diet with monounsaturated fat can lead to health benefits, including increased insulin sensitivity, better blood sugar control, and lower levels of "bad" LDL-cholesterol. It can help you feel full (because of the fat and fiber), but because avocado is relatively high in fat, it is also high in calories—about 231 calories for 3.5 oz (or 100 g). So if you're trying to lose weight, be sure to stick to reasonable portions.

RED RICE AND FRUIT PUDDING

Total preparation time: **45 minutes**
Cooking time: **40 minutes**
Yield: **2 servings**

3/4 cup (about140 g) red rice, washed under cold running water
2 ripe nectarines or 1 mango
1 tablespoon juice organic lime
1 tablespoon toasted granola hazelnuts
1 medium ripe banana
½ cup (120 ml) hazelnut milk
2 teaspoons honey
4 heaping tablespoons plain yogurt
1 pinch of cinnamon

1   In a pan, bring water to a boil. Add rice and cook for about
     40 minutes. You can speed up the process by using a pressure
     cooker (about 12 minutes). Rice should be sticky when done.
     Drain and let cool. You can prepare rice and keep it in the
     refrigerator for up to 2–3 days, which is a great time-saver.

2   Coarsely chop nectarines and place in a blender with the lime
     juice. Blend until smooth and set aside.

3   Place banana, hazelnut milk, and 2/3 of the rice in the blender.
     Blend until smooth. Transfer to a bowl and stir in the rest of
     the rice.

4   Place 1 tablespoon of yogurt in each glass and divide the
     pudding between the two glasses. Top with a layer of nectarine
     purée, then the remaining yogurt, and a pinch of cinnamon.
     Drizzle some honey and add hazelnut granola. Serve imme-
     diately. This is a great recipe for a weekend brunch, when you
     might have more time to cook and enjoy your meal.

MAMMA MIA!

Red yeast rice (RYR), commonly known as **red rice,** is a Chinese type of rice that is popular in Italy for its health benefits. The red color comes from pigments (mostly oligoketides) released by the molds used in the red yeast rice's production, which improves the rice's aesthetic appeal. It is a kind of unpolished rice with a nutty taste and a gratifying flavor that goes well with most meats and vegetables, or served as a pilaf or salad. It is high in nutritional value, being **rich in fiber, vitamins B1 and B2, iron,** and **calcium**. Its high fiber content also **helps in maintaining a healthy weight**.

Red yeast rice in **traditional Chinese medicine** has been shown **to lower cholesterol**. Several studies have shown good evidence that RYR can significantly lower total and LDL-cholesterol. RYR contains monacolin K, something similar to the active ingredient in the cholesterol-lowering drugs called **statins**. However, while supplements may be a good choice, **it is always important to ask your doctor** before taking any supplement.

WHOLE GRAIN ITALIAN BREAD

Total preparation time: **50 minutes + 2 hours for rising**
Baking time: **40 minutes**
Yield: **1 loaf, or about 2 pounds (900 g)**

2⅓ cups (330 g) whole grain wheat flour + some extra for
    kneading the dough
1½ cups (210 g) rye flour
2 tablespoons sunflower seeds
2 tablespoons sesame or flax seeds
1½ teaspoons (about 8 g) sea salt
1⅓ cups (320 ml) water at 100°F (38°C)
1 teaspoon malt or honey
1 cube (about 1 scarce oz or 23 g) fresh yeast or 1 package (1
    heaping teaspoon or 9 g) dried yeast

1   In a small pitcher, dissolve malt or honey in warm water, then
     add yeast and mix well. The sugar serves as "nourishment" for
     the yeast. Let it rest for 1–2 minutes.

2   In a large bowl, mix flours, seeds, and salt. Add water to flour
     mix. Mix well until you have a smooth and even dough that is
     still a little bit sticky.

3   Remove dough from the bowl and turn it out onto a lightly
     floured surface. Knead briefly, about 6–8 minutes, adding
     some wheat flour to work it easily. (Do not add too much
     flour, otherwise dough will get tough. The amount of flour
     depends on the water absorption capacity of flours; you might
     need 1-2 tablespoons extra.)

4   Place the dough in a glass bowl and cover with plastic wrap.
     Let rise in a warm, draft-free place (about 77°F or 25°C) for
     about 1½–2 hours, until the mixture has doubled in size.

Oatmeal and
Banana Cake
page 170

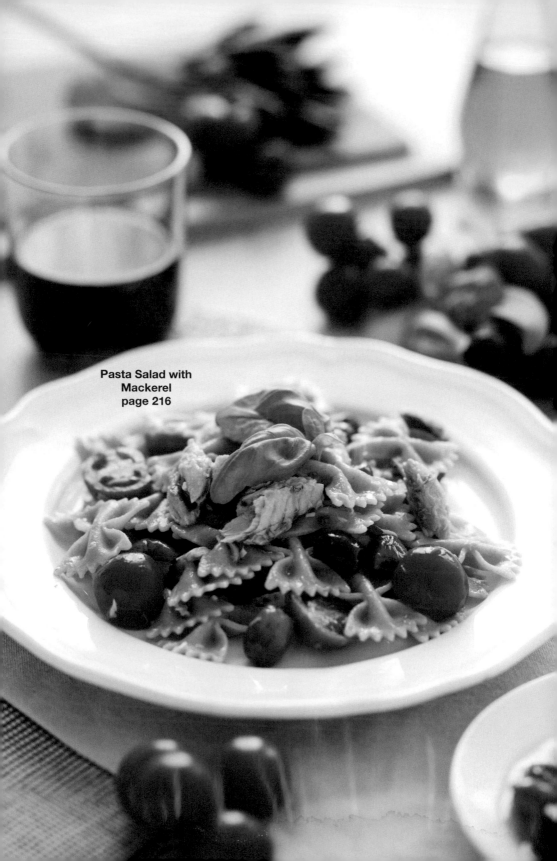

Pasta Salad with Mackerel page 216

**Marinated Chicken
Breast in Orange Juice
with Pistachios
page 270**

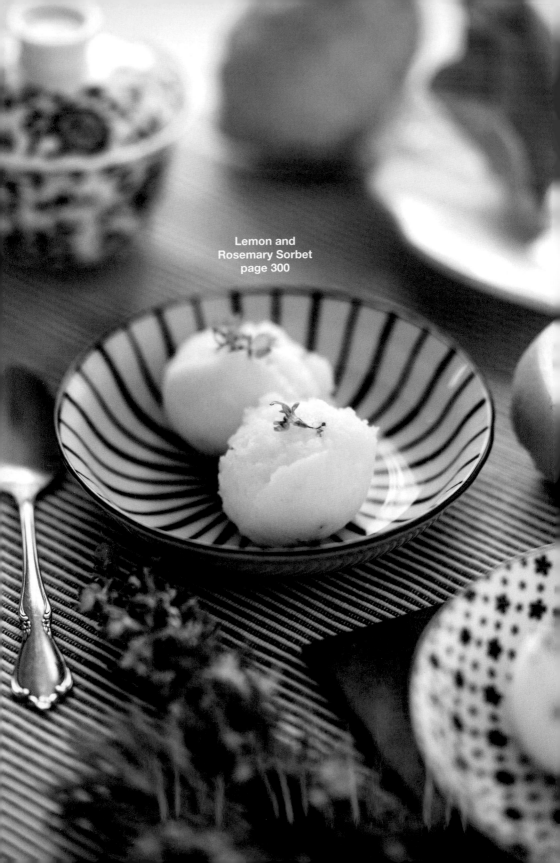

Lemon and
Rosemary Sorbet
page 300

5   Preheat the oven to 425°F (220°C). Set oven rack to middle
     position. The ideal baking method is in a vapor oven; if not
     available, add a baking pan full of water on the lower rack and
     sprinkle the dough with some drops of water.

6   Remove dough from the bowl and place into a nonstick,
     lightly oiled and floured 10 x 5 in. (25 x 12.5 cm) pan. Cover
     with plastic wrap and let rest at room temperature for about 10
     minutes.

7   Bake for 35–40 minutes. Remove from oven and let rest on a
     cooling rack for a few minutes.

8   Turn it upside down and remove from pan. Give the bottom
     of the loaf a firm *thump* with your thumb, like striking a
     drum. Bread will sound hollow when it's done. You can keep
     the bread for a few days wrapped in a kitchen towel at room
     temperature or store in in the freezer wrapped in plastic wrap.

MAMMA MIA!

Homemade rye and whole grain wheat bread is certainly a healthy choice. **Rye** is a cereal that looks like
wheat, but is longer and more slender and varies in
color. Because it is difficult to separate the germ and
bran from the endosperm of rye, rye flour usually retains
a **large quantity of nutrients and fiber**, in contrast
to refined wheat flour. It therefore has many health benefits, including managing metabolic disorder. The fiber
found in rye is also rich in non-cellulose polysaccharides
that have exceptionally high water-binding capacity,
quickly giving a feeling of fullness and satiety.

STARTERS

ARUGULA AND WALNUT SALAD

Preparation time: **10 minutes**
Yield: **2 servings**

3 oz (80 g) arugula
2 medium ripe Williams pears or Conference pears
10 walnut halves or pecans
1½ tablespoons extra virgin olive oil
Balsamic vinegar glaze
Sea salt and freshly ground pepper, to taste
Parmesan cheese or Roquefort (optional)

1 Wash arugula under cold water and dry.

2 Peel pears, cut into quarters, and remove cores. Cut each quarter in half.

3 Place arugula in one large serving dish or two individual ones. Add some pears and decorate with walnuts. Bring salt, pepper, balsamic vinegar glaze and olive oil to the table and let each diner dress his or her own salad, according to the Italian tradition.

MAMMA MIA!

This salad, made with arugula and walnuts, is a contrast of different flavors that blend well together. They create a harmonious taste that ranges from the pungent flavor of the arugula to the sweet and delicate taste of the pears to the nutty taste of walnuts. You can shave some Parmesan cheese or add some Roquefort, too; the calorie content will increase, but so will the flavor!

ITALIAN SALAD

Preparation time: **10 minutes**
Yield: **2 servings**

3 oz (80 g) spring lettuce
4 radishes, finely sliced
1–2 medium Roma tomatoes, sliced
½ medium fennel, finely sliced with a mandolin or meat slider
1 medium carrot, peeled and julienne sliced
5–6 capers preserved in salt, washed and dried
1 tablespoon toasted pumpkin seeds
2 tablespoons extra virgin olive oil
½ tablespoon balsamic vinegar
Sea salt and freshly ground pepper, to taste

1   Wash all vegetables before preparing as called for in the ingredients.

2   In a large bowl, combine all ingredients and dress according to the Italian tradition: salt first, vinegar and olive oil last.

MAMMA MIA!

Arugula, popularized centuries ago by the Romans for its supposed aphrodisiac qualities, also has digestive and diuretic properties, not to mention being rich in potassium and vitamin C.

ITALIAN-STYLE CRUDITES

Preparation time: **10 minutes**
Yield: **2 servings**

1 large carrot, peeled
1 fennel bulb
1 celery stalk, leaves trimmed
1 medium bell pepper, cut in half and seeded
1 medium cucumber, peeled
1/4 cup (60 ml) extra virgin olive oil
1 tablespoon lemon juice
3–4 basil leaves, torn into small pieces
Sea salt and freshly ground pepper, to taste

1	Wash vegetables under running water and pat dry with paper towels.

2	Slice vegetables into small sticks.

3	Arrange vegetables on a large plate, leaving some space in the center for the dip.

4	Prepare dip by mixing salt, lemon juice, olive oil , pepper and basil together with a fork in a small bowl.

5	Place the bowl in the center of the vegetable plate.

MAMMA MIA!

Italian-style crudites, called *pinzimonio*, are a healthy starter. The seasoning can also be enriched according to personal taste by choosing from lemon juice or balsamic vinegar, pepper, mustard, herbs (such as thyme, basil, chives, or parsley), and hot chili pepper. There are other vegetables which can be used depending on the season; for example, artichoke hearts, salad tomatoes, Belgian leaves, avocados, fresh onions, or red onions.

BABY SPINACH AND POMEGRANATE SALAD

Preparation time: **15 minutes**
Yield: **2 servings**

4 oz (110 g) baby spinach or Italian *songino* lettuce
1 medium ripe Williams pear or Conference pear
5–6 tablespoons pomegranate seeds
2 tablespoons walnut or pecan halves
4 oz (110 g) fresh goat cheese (for example Italian*caprino*), cut
   in pieces
Extra virgin olive oil
Freshly ground pepper, to taste

1   Wash baby spinach under cold water and dry.

2   Seed pomegranate. To clean pomegranate, use a sharp knife to halve the pomegranate across its diameter. Make a small cuts in the membrane in each pomegranate half; then, working over a bowl, start hitting the back of pomegranate with a wooden spoon. If done correctly, all the seeds should fall right out into the bowl. This method can be a little bit messy, so work gently and avoid a wooden cutting board, because pome-granate juice does stain. (You can, however, remove stains with lemon juice or white vinegar.)

3   Peel pear, cut into quarters, and remove core. Cut each quarter into four thin slices.

4   Place equal portions of baby spinach on two single plates. Arrange half the pear slices on each plate and add 2–3 table-spoons of pomegranate seeds and 1 spoonful of nuts. Place ½ of cheese on each plate. Bring olive oil and pepper to the table and let each diner dress his or her own salad according to the Italian tradition!

MAMMA MIA!

Pomegranate is certainly one of my favorite winter fruits. It is delicious whether eaten alone, used in a recipe, or enjoyed as fresh juice. It is also very healthy, a veritable **winter superfood, rich in antioxidants and nutritious compounds with anti-cancer and anti-arthritic properties. It also a good ally to your heart, and it is certainly something to add to your diet.** Pomegranate has been enjoyed for thousands of years and is a symbol of hope and abundance. I love a few kernels of it in my champagne at New Year's Eve!

Pomegranate has been part of the Mediterranean culture since prehistoric times. Its name in Italian, "melagrana," comes from Latin *malum* (*mela* meaning apple) and *granatum* (*con i semi*, with seeds).

Caprino, an Italian fresh goat cheese, is a great choice for this dish because it has less cholesterol and lactose, which may make it a better option for those who are mildly lactose intolerant. You can also substitute with any other fresh goat cheese you have available.

CAPRESE SALAD

Preparation time: **5 minutes**
Yield: **2 servings**

4 medium ripe Roma tomatoes or Heirloom tomatoes
5 oz (140 g) fresh cow mozzarella or buffalo mozzarella, at room
    temperature
2–3 tablespoons extra virgin olive oil
Basil leaves
Dried oregano, to taste
Freshly ground pepper, to taste

1   Wash tomatoes and pat dry with paper towels. Cut into slices
     ½ inch (about 1 cm) thick.

2   Remove mozzarella from the liquid and cut into slices ½ inch
     (about 1 cm) thick.

3   Place tomatoes on a serving dish. Cover with mozzarella and
     season generously with freshly ground pepper and oregano.
     Drizzle with olive oil and decorate with fresh basil leaves.
     Serve immediately.

MAMMA MIA!

Mozzarella is a fresh and soft Italian cheese with an elastic texture made from cow's or buffalo milk (which has a stronger taste). Consumption of mozzarella should be **limited to once a week.** The name mozzarella comes from *mozzatura* (cutting by hand), a procedure of separation of the curd into small balls. You can store fresh mozzarella at room temperature for up to a day or in the refrigerator for a few days. Before serving, bring the cheese to room temperature. A fast way to do this is to put it in warm water for 2–3 minutes.

FENNEL AND ORANGE SALAD

Preparation time: **15 minutes**
Yield: **2 servings**

1 medium fennel bulb, thinly shaved with a mandolin or meat
   slicer
1 medium blood or Navel orange, peeled
6 green olives or black, pitted and sliced + 4 whole pitted olives
½ teaspoon fresh lemon juice
2 tablespoons extra virgin olive oil
Sea salt and freshly ground pepper, to taste

1   Soak unpeeled oranges in boiling water for about 5 minutes.
    (This method facilitates removal of white membrane when
    peeling.)

2   Using a sharp knife, peel oranges and remove the membrane.
    Cut into the shape you prefer; I like cutting one into small
    pieces and the other one in slices.

3   Wash fennel bulbs, slicing off the stalk and any fronds, and
    slice thinly with a mandolin.

4   In a large bowl, combine orange pieces, fennel, and sliced
    olives.

5   To make the dressing, mix salt, pepper, lemon juice, and olive
    oil together in a small bowl. Toss salad with the dressing.

6   Arrange sliced oranges on a serving plate. Place salad mix in
    the middle and decorate with whole olives. Serve immediately.
    This salad is a delicious and refreshing starter and is ideal
    before a fish dish.

MAMMA MIA!

Fennel bulb, foliage, and **seeds** have been used for centuries in Italy for **culinary** and **medicinal purposes**. This salad is not only very beautiful, but it is also delightfully healthy. Fennel is **purifying, diuretic,** and **low in calories.** It is also rich in **vitamin C and antioxidants.** When purchasing your vegetables, choose fresh fennel, and select "male" (round) fennel if possible—the taste is superior. Fennel turns brown (oxidizes) rapidly, so quickly add dressing as soon as you slice it. The presence of lemon juice will slow down the process.

WATERMELON AND CELERY SALAD

Preparation time: **10 minutes**
Yield: **2 servings**

11 oz (310 g), peeled, seeded, and chilled watermelon
3 oz (80 g) *quartirolo* or feta cheese
2 stalks green celery, finely sliced
2 tablespoons Taggiasche olives or black olives, pitted
1½ tablespoons extra virgin olive oil
Freshly ground pepper, to taste

1   Cut watermelon into 1 inch (2.5 cm) chunks.

2   In a small bowl, mix celery, olives, olive oil, and a pinch of pepper.

3   In a large bowl, combine all ingredients and mix gently. Serve immediately or the watermelon will lose water. Feel free to try a variation on this salad by adding mint leaves before serving.

MAMMA MIA!

Watermelon has become synonymous with summer, and is perfect during the hot months to prevent dehydration (in fact, it is 92 percent water!) It also provides a high amount of **vitamins, minerals, and antioxidants** for a low amount of calories. And, while it's cooked tomatoes that have gotten the most press when it comes to their lycopene content, you might be surprised to hear that watermelon is also a **great source of lycopene**.

LUNCH

BEANS AND FARRO SOUP

Total preparation time: **1 hour and 10 minutes + soaking time**
Cooking time: **1 hour**
Yield: **4 servings**

10 oz (280 g) mix of different types of dried beans
⅓ cup (about 60 g) *farro medio* or spelt (refer to *Mamma Mia!*
   below)
1 medium onion, finely chopped
2 garlic cloves, finely chopped
2 medium carrots, cut into slices
2 celery stalks, sliced
1 bay leaf
1 sprig thyme
2 sage leaves
4 tablespoons extra virgin olive oil
2 tomatoes, peeled and diced
3 tablespoons tomato sauce
Parmesan rind (1–2 pieces), optional
Sea salt and freshly ground pepper, to taste

1   In a large bowl, soak beans for at least 6 hours (see instruction
     on the package). Drain, and then place in a large pan with the
     bay leaf and cover with cold water. Bring to a boil and cook,
     covered, over medium-low heat for about 30 minutes. Drain,
     remove bay leaf, and set aside.

2   In a saucepan over medium-low heat, sauté onion, garlic,
     carrot, and celery in olive oil for a few minutes. Add beans.
     Mix and cook over high heat for a few minutes, stirring with a
     wooden spoon.

3   Add tomatoes, tomato sauce and fresh herbs. Cover with plenty of water before covering with a lid and cooking for about 10 minutes.

4   Add farro (previously washed under cold water) and Parmesan rind (scraped with a knife, washed and dried). Complete cooking for about 20 minutes until all vegetables are tender and farro is *al dente* (the exact cooking time for legumes and farro should be indicated on the packages). Remove herbs.

5   Add salt and freshly ground pepper to taste. Cook for 1–2 minutes. You can top this soup with some grated Parmesan cheese or, if you prefer, you can sprinkle some hot chili olive oil before serving.

MAMMA MIA!

Spelt or **farro**? There is some confusion. **Spelt** (*Triticum spelta*), **emmer** (*Triticum dicoccum*), and **einkorn** (*Triticum monococcum*), are collectively called *farro* in Italy. Sometimes, but not always, they will be distinguished as *farro grande* (big), *farro medio* (medium), and *farro piccolo* (small), respectively. **Emmer (farro medio) is typical of Tuscany and mainly used in Italy.** It is one of the oldest cultivated crops in human history and is believed to have first been used between 7,000 and 8,000 years ago. Farro is rich in protein, fiber, vitamins and minerals. It has a lot of health benefits, including **regulating the body's metabolism, lowering blood sugar, reducing cholesterol levels,** and **boosting digestive function.** It *does* contain gluten, so I would suggest **brown rice for a gluten-free version**.

BUCKWHEAT PASTA WITH PRAWNS AND SPINACH

Total preparation time: **15 minutes**
Cooking time: **8 minutes**
Yield: **2 servings**

5 oz (140 g) buckwheat *penne* (or any other short, gluten-free
    pasta)
6 oz (170 g) fresh spinach leaves, cleaned and cut in small strips
10–12 prawns, cleaned and de-veined
1–2 garlic cloves
2 tablespoons extra virgin olive oil
Sea salt and freshly ground pepper, to taste

1   In a large pot, bring to boil a generous amount of salted water.
    Add pasta and cook until *al dente*—about 7–8 minutes (the
    exact cooking time will be indicated on the package).

2   While pasta is cooking, heat olive oil in a nonstick pan and
    sauté garlic over medium heat until lightly browned (but
    not burnt). Remove and add spinach. Cook for 3–4 minutes,
    stirring. Add prawns and cook for 3–4 minutes (until just
    pinkish-red but not overcooked), stirring a few times.

3   Drain pasta, reserving ¼ scarce cup (50 ml) of cooking water,
    and add to the sauce. Add pasta and toss gently over high heat.
    Place on a serving dish and flavor with some freshly ground
    pepper. Serve immediately.

MAMMA MIA!

Buckwheat is not a cereal grain (as most people think); it is actually a fruit related to rhubarb and sorrel. Because its seeds are edible and rich in complex carbohydrates, it is referred to as a pseudo-cereal. It is **gluten-free** and makes a suitable substitute for people who are sensitive to wheat or other grains containing gluten. It also has a low Glycemic Index. Buckwheat is packed with protein, fiber, minerals, vitamins, and bio-active compounds (flavonoids); it has even been linked to **reducing LDL cholesterol levels** and maintaining **healthy blood pressure.**

CHICKEN BREAST "PIZZAIOLA"

Total preparation time: **20 minutes**
Cooking time: **15 minutes**
Yield: **2 servings**

10 oz (280 g) chicken breast
½ medium shallot, finely chopped
3 tablespoons extra virgin olive oil
½ ladle warm water
1½ cups (about 300 g) canned cherry tomatoes
¼ cup (60 ml) dry white wine
2–3 tablespoons all-purpose flour
1 teaspoon dried oregano
2 tablespoons capers preserved in salt, washed and dried
½ teaspoon chili pepper flakes
Sea salt, to taste

1   In a pan, heat 1 tablespoon of olive oil. Add shallot and sauté
    for 1 minute over medium-low heat. Add water and continue
    cooking for an additional 3 minutes.

2   Add tomatoes, oregano, capers, and chili pepper. Cook for 10
    minutes over medium heat.

3   While sauce is cooking, flour the chicken breast. If you want to
    make this recipe lighter, you can avoid this step by cutting the
    chicken breast into cubes and adding directly to the sauce.

4   In a nonstick pan, heat 2 tablespoons olive oil and sauté
    chicken on both side over medium heat. Add wine and let it
    evaporate. Cook for a few minutes—just enough to brown the
    meat.

5   Add chicken breast to the tomato sauce. Cover with a lid and
    cook for 2–3 minutes over medium-low heat. Remove the

lid, add a pinch of salt, and cook for 5 additional minutes at medium-high heat to concentrate the sauce. Serve warm with steamed brown rice (1 serving is equal to ½ scarce cup or 70 g) and some steamed green beans.

MAMMA MIA!

Chili pepper (Capsicum annum), the mysterious spice with **stimulating, vasodilating, and aphrodisiac properties,** was brought to Europe by Christopher Columbus from America, where it was used by the natives going back to ancient times (5,500 BCE). Today, it is one the main spices in Mediterranean cuisine and is used especially in Italy's southern regions to prepare various recipes, adding flavor and spiciness to many dishes. In fact, the name Capsicum seems to have come from the Greek word "kapto" (to bite), referring to one biting his tongue because the strong taste. For more health benefits of chili pepper, refer to page 153.

PASTA WITH EGGPLANT

Total preparation time: **1 hour**
Cooking time: **10–12 minutes**
Yield: **2 servings**

5 oz (140 g) spaghetti or linguine
1 medium eggplant
2 garlic cloves
9 oz (250 g) tomato sauce
4 tablespoons extra virgin olive oil
2 tablespoons grated ricotta cheese
Fresh basil leaves
Kosher salt and freshly ground pepper, to taste

1   Wash eggplant under cold water. Cut off ends and slice vertically into 3/8 inch (or 8 mm) thick slices. Arrange a single layer of slices in the bottom of a large colander and sprinkle with kosher salt. Repeat this procedure until all of eggplant slices are in the colander.

2   Weigh down slices with something heavy (for example, three or four plates) and let drain for 40–50 minutes. This helps release some of the moisture before cooking. Brush off the salt and dry well on paper towels. Cut slices into ½ in (1 cm) cubes.

3   In a large nonstick pan, heat 3 tablespoons oil olive over medium heat. Add eggplant cubes and cook, tossing occasionally, until golden brown. Remove from pan and place on paper towel to remove excess oil.

4   Bring a large pot of salted water to boil and cook pasta *al dente* (according to the instructions on the package).

5   While pasta is cooking, sauté garlic in a large nonstick pan
    in 1 tablespoon of olive oil over medium heat until lightly
    browned, then remove. Add tomato sauce and pepper to taste.
    Cook for 5 minutes and then add eggplant. Cook for 1 minute
    to mix the flavors.

6   Drain pasta, reserving 2 tablespoons of cooking water to add
    to the sauce Add cooking water and toss gently. Season with
    basil and ricotta cheese and serve immediately.

MAMMA MIA!

This dish calls to mind all the flavor and tradition of
beautiful Sicily, the land of sun and extraordinary culinary culture. This recipe is called *Pasta alla Norma* in
Italian and is dedicated to the famous opera *La Norma*,
composed by Sicilian musician Vincenzo Bellini.

LINGUINE WITH CLAM

Total preparation time: **15–20 minutes**
Cooking time: **11–12 minutes**
Yield: **2 servings**

5 oz (140 g) linguine pasta
6 oz (170 g) canned claims
2 tablespoons extra virgin olive oil
1 garlic clove
7 oz (200 g) fresh tomatoes, finely chopped
1 teaspoon fresh parsley, finely chopped
Sea salt and freshly ground pepper, to taste

1   Bring a large pot of salted water to boil and cook pasta *al dente* (according to the instructions on the package).

2   While pasta is cooking, sauté garlic in olive oil in a large nonstick pan over medium heat until lightly browned, and then remove. Add chopped tomatoes and half the clam liquid. Cook over medium-low heat until sauce begins to thicken (about 8–10 minutes). One minute before pasta is ready, add parsley and clams to the sauce.

3   Drain pasta, reserving 2 tablespoons of cooking water to add to the sauce. Add cooking water and toss gently. Season with pepper to taste and serve immediately.

MAMMA MIA!

Clams are mollusks popular in the Italian cuisine. The most commonly used are *vongole* and *cozze*. Clams are nutrient-dense, containing many vitamins and minerals. They are considered a lean protein choice because they are low in fat while still being packed with a lot of protein and iron.

CHICKPEA SALAD

Total preparation time: **60 minutes + soaking time**
Cooking time: **50–60 minutes**
Yield: **2 servings**

½ cup (100 g) dried chickpeas
1 bay leaf
½ pound (225 g) cherry tomatoes
½ medium purple onion, finely sliced
2 tablespoons Taggiasche olives or black olives, pitted
2.5 oz (70 g) *quartirolo* or feta cheese, diced
½ tablespoon fresh lemon juice
1½ tablespoons extra virgin olive oil
Fresh basil leaves
Sea salt and freshly ground pepper, to taste

1   In a large bowl, soak chickpeas for at least 6 hours (see instruction on the package). Drain and place in a large pan with a bay leaf, covering with cold water. Bring to a boil, and cook covered over medium-low heat for about 50–60 minutes. Drain, rinse under cold water, remove and discharge bay leaf, and set aside. To save time you can use canned chickpeas (about 1 heaping cup, or 240 g). If doing so, drain chickpeas using a colander and rinse under cold running water until no more foam appears.

2   Remove the skin. Add lemon juice and set aside.

3   Cut tomatoes, add some salt, and let them rest for 10 minutes.

4   Drain tomatoes in a colander. Slice the onion and tear the basil by hand. In a large bowl, mix together with the olives, chickpeas, and olive oil.

5   Add cheese to vegetable mix.

6   Season with salt, if necessary, and pepper to taste. Let the salad
    rest for 10 minutes and serve at room temperature with rustic
    bread (1 serving is equivalent to 1 slice).

MAMMA MIA!

Chickpeas—or garbanzo beans—are **legumes,
rich in protein, minerals (magnesium, potassium, iron), vitamin A, folate, and fiber, and
low in fat** (most of which are PUFAs). Chickpeas are
one of the earliest cultivated legumes: remains have
been found in the Middle East dating back almost 7,500
years. They are largely cultivated in the Mediterranean
area and are well known in Italian cuisine.

Quartirolo is an Italian cow's milk cheese with a
lower fat content compared to cheddar that goes well
with salads, walnuts and honey. You can easily substitute
with feta cheese, which has a stronger taste.

FARRO "LINGUINE" WITH LEEKS AND NUTS

Total preparation time: **15 minutes**
Cooking time: **10–12 minutes**
Yield: **2 servings**

5 oz (140 g) *farro* or spelt linguine
2 medium leeks, cleaned and finely sliced
15 walnut halves, coarsely chopped
2 tablespoons extra virgin olive oil
2 tablespoons grated Parmesan cheese (optional)
Sea salt and freshly ground pepper, to taste

1   In a large pot, bring to a boil plenty of water, lightly salted, and
    cook pasta *al dente* (the exact cooking time will be indicated
    on the package).

2   While pasta is cooking, wash leeks under cold running water.
    Clean by removing the green part and finely slice.

3   In a nonstick pan, heat olive oil over medium heat. Add leeks
    and cook for a few minutes, mixing with a wooden spoon.
    After 3 minutes, add 2–3 tablespoons of water and cook until
    soft. Add nuts and mix well, turning the heat to low to keep it
    warm. Add salt and pepper to taste.

4   Drain pasta, reserving about scarce ¼ cup (50 ml) of cooking
    water, and add pasta to the leeks. Add cooking water and toss
    gently over high heat.

5   Place pasta on a serving plate, sprinkle with grated Parmesan
    cheese (optional), and serve immediately.

MAMMA MIA!

Leeks belong to the Allium genus, along with onion, shallots and garlic. These are the ancient **superfoods** used in the Egyptian cuisine as early as the second millennium BCE, both as vegetables and as aromatic herbs. In Roman times, Emperor Nero is known to have loved leeks in his soups, believing they improved the resonance of his voice. Leeks are nutritious and healthy, rich in water (over 90 percent) and fiber, and contain moderate amounts of B vitamins and folate. Leeks also contain the flavonoid **kaempferol**, which acts to neutralize free radicals and superoxide radicals in the body, as well as preserve the activities of various antioxidant enzymes. It has even been shown to have platelet anti-aggregation activity, meaning leeks provide cardiovascular benefits.

HOMEMADE "TAGLIATELLE" WITH PEAS AND ASPARAGUS

Total preparation time: **45 minutes**
Cooking time: **10 minutes**
Yield: **2 servings**

7 oz (200 g) fresh *tagliatelle* pasta or 5 oz (140 g) dried *tagliatelle*
    pasta
Homemade Fresh Tagliatelle
1½ cups (about 200 g) Italian flour Grade 00 or all-purpose
    flour + extra flour for kneading
2 medium eggs, at room temperature
Sauce
1 cup (150 g) fresh peas
10 asparagus spears, cut into 1½ inch (about 4 cm) chunks
6 fresh basil leaves, torn into pieces
½ medium shallot, finely chopped
2 tablespoons extra virgin olive oil
2/3 cup vegetable stock
2 tablespoons grated Parmesan cheese
Sea salt and freshly ground pepper, to taste

1   If time is a factor, you can buy dried *tagliatelle* in most super-
markets. However, I'll always prefer using fresh pasta whenever possible—and it's so much fun to make! Place flour in a
volcano-shaped pile on a work surface (wood is the traditional
material) or in a large bowl, making sure that the "crater"
provides a large enough well in the center to receive the eggs.

2   Wash eggs under running water, pat dry, and crack into the
well. Beat eggs with a fork for 1–2 minutes, and then gradually
blend flour into the eggs, starting from the inner wall of the

well and continuing until flour and eggs are completely combined. Add flour until the dough is no longer sticky (you may
have to use extra flour depending on the absorption characteristics of the flour and the temperature of the room).

3   Knead dough for about 10–15 minutes to form a smooth,
     elastic ball.

4   Place dough on a clean cotton dish towel or plastic wrap and
     let rest for about 20 minutes at room temperature.

5   Divide your pasta in four equal parts and roll each one out,
     one part at a time (keeping the rest on the dish towel until
     ready to work). Use a wooden rolling pin. Dust each piece
     lightly with flour and roll out to the desired thickness, which
     should be pretty thin (1/16 inch, or about 1.5 mm). Work
     quickly, because pasta dries much quicker than you might
     think.

6   Starting with the short end, gently fold the dried sheet at 2
     inch (5 cm) intervals to create a flat, rectangular roll. Cut the
     dough into 3/16-inch-thick (about 5 mm) *tagliatelle* with a
     sharp knife. Using your fingers, unfurl the pasta and transfer
     to a floured cotton towel.

PREPARING THE SAUCE

1   While pasta is resting, prepare sauce. Heat olive oil in a sauce-
     pan and gently sauté shallot on medium-low heat until soft.

2   Add peas and cook for 1–2 minutes at medium heat. Add
     stock and pepper. Cover, then cook over medium-low heat
     for about 10 minutes. They should be tender, but not soft. The
     right cooking time it depends on the size of the peas and the
     thickness of their skin. If you're using frozen peas, cook for 5
     minutes with half of the stock.

3   Add asparagus and continue cooking without a lid until most
     of the liquid has evaporated. A few minutes before removing
     from the heat, add salt and basil. The asparagus should be
     crisp. Keep warm.

4   In a large pot, bring to boil plenty of salted water. Add fresh
     pasta and cook *al dente* for 3–4 minutes.

5   Drain pasta, reserving about 2 tablespoons of the cooking
     water. Add pasta to the vegetable sauce. Add cooking water
     and toss gently.

6   Place pasta on a serving plate and serve immediately with
     Parmesan cheese.

ROLLING OUT BY MACHINE

While you can certainly roll pasta by hand or using a
wooden pin, a hand-cranked pasta machine is the best
to use. Kids especially love turning the crank and seeing
the pasta come out! Start out using the widest setting
and run the pasta through about 4–5 times, until the
dough is smooth. If the sheet tears, dust it with flour.

Continue to run each sheet through the machine,
reducing the thickness a notch at a time, until you reach
the desired thickness of about 4–5 for *tagliatelle* (1/16
inch or about 1.5 mm, usually notch 4 or 5 out of 7).
Cut the pasta into rectangular sheets (10 x 4 in.) and let
them rest for a few minutes on a cotton dish towel. Then
use the *tagliattelle* setting and dry your fresh *tagliatelle*
on a pasta drying rack.

MAMMA MIA!

Asparagus is native to the Mediterranean area. Asparagus comes in different colors and varieties: white asparagus (which has a delicate flavor); violet (which has a fruity taste); and green (known for having a sweeter taste). In my recipes, I mainly use the violet and the green varieties.

Asparagus, which belongs to the same family as garlic and onion, shares the same natural **diuretic properties** as its siblings. It is therefore a great ally in removing toxins and keeping your body clean. In addition, it is rich in antioxidants. This, along with its ability to neutralize cell-damaging free radicals and slow the aging process, makes it one of the top ranked vegetables in terms of health benefits.

Peas, like all legumes, are little **powerhouses** of nutrition—**low in fat and rich in protein, fiber, and micronutrients**.

LENTIL SALAD

Total preparation time: **30 minutes + soaking time**
Cooking time: **20 minutes**
Yield: **2 servings**

2/3 cup (140 g) dried green or red lentils
1 bay leaf
5 oz (140 g) cherry tomatoes
½ medium cucumber, diced
½ medium red onion, diced
½ medium bell pepper, diced
1 tablespoon Taggiasche olives or black olives, pitted
1 bunch basil
2 tablespoons extra virgin olive oil
Sea salt and freshly ground pepper, to taste

1   In a large bowl, soak lentils for at least 2–3 hours (see
    instructions on the package), changing water once or twice.
    (If you don't have time, you can also cook lentils straight away
    without soaking.)

2   Rinse lentils under running water, place in a pan with bay leaf
    and plenty of water, and bring to boil. Cook on medium-low
    heat, covered with a lid, until lentils are crisp, about 18–20
    minutes. A few minutes before they are done, add some salt.
    Drain and allow to cool.

3   While lentils are cooking, cut tomatoes in half and dice
    cucumber. Mix in a bowl with a pinch of salt and let stand for
    about 15 minutes at room temperature to remove excessive
    water.

4   Drain tomatoes and cucumber with a strainer. Dice onion and
    bell pepper. In a large bowl, mix all vegetables together.

5   In a small bowl, prepare a dressing using olive oil, salt and pepper.

6   Add lentils and some basil leaves to the vegetable mix and toss with the dressing. Let rest at room temperature for 10 minutes and serve at room temperature. You can keep this dish in the refrigerator for up to two days. This dish makes for a perfect lunch box, and can be enjoyed with whole grain bread (1 serving is equivalent to 1 slice).

MAMMA MIA!

Lentils, like all legumes, are an important **nutritional source of protein and good carbohydrates.** In the past they were known as "la carne dei poveri" (the meat of poor people), but they are also low in fat. In fact, lentils have a marvelous **nutritional profile**: Thirty percent of their energy comes from **protein**, with the remainder coming primarily from high quality **resistant starch**, a carbohydrate which passes the length of the gastrointestinal tract and acts as dietary fiber. This type of starch is filling, **reduces cholesterol**, and **increases fatty acids metabolism**. It also encourages **healthy intestinal bacteria growth** by providing butyrate as selective fuel. These bacteria protect against cancers of the gastrointestinal tract, as they have anti-carcinogenic and anti-inflammatory effects. Lentils are also **rich in potassium, phosphorus, calcium, and magnesium.**

MEDITERRANEAN SALAD

Preparation time: **30 minutes**
Cooking time: **20 minutes**
Yield: **2 servings**

Mixed lettuce for garnish
2 medium potatoes
6 oz (170 g) green beans, cleaned (ends removed) and washed
6 oz (170 g) cherry tomatoes
½ medium cucumber, peeled and sliced
½ medium red onion, peeled and sliced into thin rings
2 hard-boiled eggs
4 oz (110 g) canned tuna in olive oil (drained) or fresh grilled
   tuna
Taggiasche or black olives, pitted, to taste
Capers preserved in salt, washed and dried, to taste
2 tablespoons extra virgin olive oil
4–5 fresh basil leaves
Salt and freshly ground pepper, to taste

1   Wash lettuce and tomatoes under cold water. Dry and set
    aside.

2   In a large pan over medium heat, cook whole potatoes in
    salted water for about 20–25 minutes. The cooking time will
    vary according to the size of the potatoes. They should be
    tender but not crumbly. Drain and allow to cool. Peel and cut
    each potato into 10–12 pieces.

3   Blanch green beans in water or steam for 6–7 minutes. They
    should be crisp. Remove beans from boiling water and
    submerge them in a cold water bath until they are cold to the
    touch, about 3 minutes. Remove and set aside.

4   Boil eggs in a saucepan covered with water for about 7–8 minutes (counting the minutes as the water begins to boil). Drain and place in cold water to cool. Remove shell and let cool completely. Cut each into four wedges.

5   You can prepare two individual plates or one large salad to serve at the table. Arrange the lettuce on the plate, then add green beans, cherry tomatoes (cut in half), potatoes, onion, cucumber, eggs, tuna, olives, and capers. Season with olive oil, a pinch of salt (optional), and pepper. Serve immediately.

MAMMA MIA!

This salad can be served as a main course for lunch on a hot day, when we most appreciate a light and refreshing meal. The addition of boiled potatoes makes this dish nutritionally complete, giving the right amount of complex carbohydrates.

We don't often think of **green beans** as providing us with of carotenoids **(potent antioxidants)** because of their green color, which is due to chlorophyll, but rest assured—they do!

PASTA SALAD WITH MACKEREL

Total preparation time: **30 minutes**
Cooking time: **11–12 minutes**
Yield: **2 servings**

3.5 oz (100 g) whole durum wheat bow-tie pasta
5 oz (140 g) cherry tomatoes
2 garlic cloves, cut in half
10–15 basil leaves
5 oz (140 g) canned mackerel, in extra virgin olive oil
2 tablespoons Taggiasche olives or black olives, pitted
1 tablespoon extra virgin olive oil, seasoned with hot chili
    pepper
Sea salt, to taste

1   Wash cherry tomatoes and cut in half. Place in a bowl with
    garlic and add a pinch of salt. Let rest for 5 minutes to release
    the water.

2   Remove garlic and drain water from tomatoes.

3   Bring a large pot of salted water to boil and cook pasta *al dente*
    for about 11–12 minutes, according to the instructions on the
    package.

4   In a bowl, mix drained and cut pieces of mackerel, tomatoes,
    and olives. Shred basil leaves by hand and add.

5   Drain pasta *al dente* and rinse with cold water. Add to the mix.
    Toss with 2 tablespoons of olive oil and serve at room tem-
    perature. You can store this dish in the refrigerator in a sealed
    container for 1 day. It is a delicious lunch box dish for summer.

MAMMA MIA!

This pasta salad is a tasty summer dish, perfect to prepare on a warm day when you don't want to stand in front of the stove but still want to enjoy a simple, refreshing and light dish! I suggest having it as a main dish for your midday meal—it is satisfying, quick and easy to prepare and rich in many nutrients. You can also prepare it for a picnic or have it for lunch at work.

Mackerels (called in Italian "pesce azzurro", like sardines or anchovies) is common in the Mediterranean sea and Is a good source of omega-3 fatty acids, minerals, and protein.

PASTA WITH BROCCOLI

Total preparation time: **25 minutes**
Cooking time: **20 minutes**
Yield: **2 servings**

1 pound (450 g) broccoli, chopped into small pieces
5 oz (140 g) whole durum wheat *penne* or any other short pasta
2 tablespoons extra virgin olive oil
1–2 garlic cloves
1 fresh hot chili peppers, seeded and finely sliced
2 salted anchovies, rinsed and coarsely chopped
2 tablespoons grated pecorino cheese
Sea salt, to taste

1   Trim away broccoli stalk, reserving florets, and wash. Cut florets into 2 inches (5 cm) pieces.

2   In a large pot, bring to boil plenty of water and just a pinch of salt (anchovies are already salty). Add broccoli and cook about 5–6 minutes. Remove broccoli with a fine mesh strainer and set aside. Don't overcook.

3   Bring broccoli water back to boil and add pasta. Cook for about 11–12 minutes (until *al dente;* the exact cooking time will be indicated on the package).

4   While pasta is cooking, in a large skillet over medium-low heat, sauté garlic, chili peppers, and chopped anchovies in olive oil for 1 minute. Mix in broccoli and sauté for 2 minutes, stirring constantly and gently to mix. Remove garlic. Add salt to taste.

5   Drain pasta, reserving about ¼ cup (60 ml) of cooking water. Add pasta to vegetable mix. Add cooking water and toss gently over high heat.

6   Place on a serving plate. Sprinkle with some grated pecorino
    cheese (optional). Serve immediately.

MAMMA MIA!

Broccoli is a superfood that supplies **loads of nutrients with few calories**. Many studies have suggested
that increased consumption of broccoli **decreases the
risk of obesity, cardiovascular disease, and
cancer.** The anti-cancer properties of broccoli have
being attributed to **selenographer**, a compound also
found in Brussels sprouts and cabbage. It is better to eat
raw broccoli to preserve all the nutrients (especially glucosinolates), so in cases where a recipe calls for cooked
broccoli, boil for a short time instead.

PASTA WITH KALE

Total preparation time: **30 minutes**
Cooking time: **20 minutes**
Yield: **2 servings**

5 oz (140 g) whole durum wheat *fusilli or penne* (any short
   pasta)
½ pound (225 g) kale or ⅓ pound (150 g), already cleaned
¼ medium white onion, finely chopped
2 tablespoons extra virgin olive oil
2/3 cup (about 200 g) creamy cow's milk ricotta cheese
1 tablespoon fresh milk
Salt and freshly ground pepper, to taste

1   Clean and wash kale and coarsely chop leaves into strips of
    about 1 inch (2.5 cm). Remove stalks.

2   In a nonstick pan, heat oil and sauté onion over medium-low
    heat. Add kale and cook over medium heat for about 5 min-
    utes, stirring occasionally. Add 2 tablespoons of water, a pinch
    of salt if desired, and pepper. Cook for another 5–8 minutes
    until kale is tender.

3   In a bowl, mix ricotta with milk until creamy.

4   While sauce is cooking, in a large pot bring to boil plenty of
    salt water. Add pasta and cook until *al dente,* about 11–12 min-
    utes (the exact cooking time will be indicated on the package).

5   Add ricotta to the kale mix, stirring to blend the flavors. Heat
    over medium heat to warm.

6   Drain pasta, reserving a ladle's worth of cooking water, and
    add to the sauce. Add cooking water. Season with freshly
    ground pepper and serve immediately.

MAMMA MIA!

Kale is a typical Tuscan vegetable that appears in the markets from October until April. Its leaves have a deep green color and a flavor that goes well with ricotta, a very delicate cheese. In addition to being delicious, **kale is rich in vitamins (pro-vitamin A, vitamin K, and vitamin C) and minerals like calcium and potassium.** Kale is among the most **nutrient-rich foods** available, and with its incredibly low calorie content, it's a surefire addition to any diet. Eating more kale is a great way to increase the total nutrient content of your diet.

RICOTTA CHEESE AND TOMATO SANDWICH

Preparation time: **5 minutes**
Yield: **2 servings**

4 medium whole grain bread slices (refer to *Whole Grain Italian Bread on page 178*)
2 lettuce leaves, washed and pat-dried
2 large Heirloom tomatoes or Roma tomatoes, cut into slices about ½ inch (about 1 cm) thick
7 oz (200 g) goat's milk ricotta cheese, sliced
2–3 fresh basil leaves
Dried oregano, to taste
Freshly ground pepper, to taste
Extra virgin olive oil

1   Place one lettuce leaf on each of the four bread slices. Add one ricotta slice, 2–3 tomato slices, a few drops of olive oil, one basil leaf, some dried oregano, and some pepper to taste.

2   Cover each slice with a slice of bread. Serve immediately.

MAMMA MIA!

Ricotta (meaning "recooked") is a typical Italian cheese made from cow, sheep, goat, and buffalo milk whey left over from the production of cheese. It is made by coagulating the protein that remains after the casein has been used to make cheese. Ricotta is one of my favorite cheeses because it has a creamy texture and slight sweet taste. It is a low fat cheese and is suitable for many recipes, both savory and sweet. I make an irresistible cheesecake with it!

SMOKE SALMON AND GRILLED ZUCCHINI SANDWICH

Preparation time: **5 minutes**
Yield: **2 servings**

2 medium zucchini
4 medium whole grain bread slices (refer to *Whole Grain Italian Bread on page 178*)
7 oz (200 g) smoked salmon
Freshly ground pepper, to taste
Homemade Cheese with Strained Yogurt
1 quart (1 liter) plain whole milk yogurt
1 pinch of sea salt
1 large piece of cheesecloth or gauze

1   Before preparing this recipe, prepare the homemade cheese with strained yogurt, if using. Place a colander over a deep bowl and line with cheesecloth. Mix yogurt with a pinch of salt and spoon it into the cheesecloth. Gather the edges up tightly and tie into a knot on top. Let it rest at slightly below room temperature for about 10–12 hours. Remove cheese from the cheesecloth and place in a closed container. Store in the fridge for up to 4–5 days. (You can also use the whey for smoothies and cakes, substituting for water.)

2   Wash zucchini under cold water. Pat dry and cut into 4–5 strips. Heat a heavy-based griddle until very hot—this can take a few minutes. Add zucchini and cook for 2–3 minutes, turning once.

3   Spread the two bread slices with 1 tablespoon each of cheese yogurt.

4   Add some pepper, three strips of grilled zucchini, and salmon, and cover with one slice of bread. If you have some zucchini leftover, you can enjoy it as a side dish with some drops of olive oil and a pinch of salt and pepper.

MAMMA MIA!

Homemade cheese with strained yogurt is tasty, light and healthy. It is also nutritious because of its high concentration of beneficial bacteria for the intestine. It can also be used by people intolerant to lactose, as **yogurt's live cultures convert lactose to lactic acid.** It is versatile, too—you can enjoy it at breakfast, lunch, or dinner with both sweet and savory dishes. You can use it as a spread on sandwiches, or serve it as a tasty appetizer, seasoned with extra virgin olive oil, olives, and oregano. You can also flavor it with fennel seeds, parsley, mint, paprika, or cumin, as you like. It makes a nice side dish with honey and mint to serve with spicy food.

SPAGHETTI WITH SARDINES AND CHERRY TOMATOES

Total preparation time: **12 minutes**
Cooking time: **10 minutes**
Yield: **2 servings**

5 oz (140 g) durum wheat spaghetti pasta
2 tablespoons extra virgin olive oil
2 garlic cloves
10–12 cherry tomatoes, halved
2 tablespoons capers preserved in salt, washed and dried
1 pinch chili pepper flakes
8 canned sardine fillets, de-boned, washed and pat dried
1 teaspoon fresh parsley, finely chopped
½ organic lemon zest
Salt, to taste

1 In a large pot, bring to boil plenty of water, lightly salted (as canned sardines are already pretty salty). Add spaghetti and cook until *al dente* (the exact cooking time will be indicated on the package).

2 In a nonstick pan, heat olive oil and sauté garlic over medium heat until golden browned (but not burnt). Remove garlic and add tomatoes, capers, and chili pepper. Cook over medium heat for 4–5 minutes.

3 Remove sardines from the can and pat dry with paper towels to remove excess oil. Add sardines and parsley to the sauce and cook for 2 minutes.

4   Drain pasta *al dente*, reserving ¼ scarce cup (50 ml) of cook-
    ing water, and add to the sauce. Add cooking water and toss
    gently over high heat. Place on a serving dish and sprinkle
    with lemon zest. Serve immediately.

MAMMA MIA!

Sardines are named after the Italian island of Sardinia.
While they are delightful when enjoyed fresh, they are
also commonly found canned. Sardines belong to the
"pesce azzurro" group and are very **rich in omega-3
fatty acids,** which are linked to **lower levels of bad
cholesterol and promote cardiovascular health**.
They are also **packed with protein**.

PASTA "ARRABBIATA"

Total preparation time: **15 minutes**
Cooking time: **11–12 minutes**
Yield: **2 servings**

5 oz (140 g) *penne* pasta
1 tablespoon extra-virgin olive oil
2 garlic cloves
1 hot chili pepper
½ teaspoon of dried hot chili pepper flakes
6 oz (170 g) tomatoes canned, diced
1 teaspoon fresh parsley, finely chopped
2 tablespoons grated pecorino cheese
Sea salt, to taste

1   Bring plenty of salted water to boil and cook pasta *al dente* (according to the instructions on the package).

2   In a saucepan, heat olive oil over medium heat. Add one garlic clove and sauté until lightly browned (not burned), and then remove.

3   Add chili pepper and turn the heat down to medium-low. Cook for 1 minute, then add tomatoes and one minced garlic clove. Cook for 8–10 minutes.

4   Drain pasta, reserving 2 tablespoons of cooking water to add to the sauce. Add cooking water and parsley. Toss gently and season with pecorino cheese. Serve immediately.

MAMMA MIA!

Pasta "arrabbiata" (or "angry" pasta) is a typical first course belonging to the Roman culinary tradition. The name is unique, harkening back to how eating chili peppers makes you red in the face, like when you're angry. It is not only very easy and fast to make, but devilishly delicious, too! The amount of chili pepper varies from person to person; what I've included here is my preference.

SPAGHETTI WITH TOMATO SAUCE AND BASIL

Total preparation time: **35 minutes**
Cooking time: **25 minutes**
Yield: **2 servings**

5 oz (140 g) whole durum wheat or durum wheat spaghetti
    pasta
Tomato Sauce
12.5 oz (350 g) ripe *S.Marzano* or Roma tomatoes, coarsely
    chopped
1–2 garlic cloves
2 tablespoons extra virgin olive oil
Fresh basil leaves
Sea salt, to taste

1   Place tomatoes in a bowl and add a pinch of salt. Let rest for
     5 minutes and then drain the liquid. Your sauce will be dense
     and tasty.

2   In a heavy saucepan, sauté e garlic in 1 tablespoon of olive oil
     until light browned (but not burned). Remove, adding toma-
     toes and some fresh basil leaves. Cook for about 10 minutes
     over medium heat, and then 15 minutes covered with a lid.
     Add a pinch of salt according to taste.

3   While sauce is cooking, bring to boil plenty of salted water and
     cook the spaghetti *al dente* according to the instructions on
     the package.

4   Pour tomato sauce into a food mill over a large bowl. Let drain
     for 2–3 minutes and discharge the liquid. Purée tomatoes until
     just the skin remains in the bowl of the food mill. This can be
     stored for 2–3 days in the refrigerator.

5   In a saucepan, heat 1 tablespoon of olive and add sauce.

6   Drain pasta, reserving 1–2 tablespoons of cooking water, and
     add to the sauce when it starts bubbling. Add cooking water
     and some basil leaves, and toss gently. Serve immediately.

MAMMA MIA!

When you purchase **tomatoes,** check to make sure that
they are firm, very red and ripe. In Italy, the best time to
buy is in July and August—those hot, sunny months when
the warmth of the summer sun brings out the full flavor
and richness of the tomatoes.

Although originating in South America, tomatoes
(called *pomodori* or "golden apples" in Italian) have
become a staple in Italian cuisine since their introduction
in the 16*th* century. **Tomatoes are rich in lycopene,**
which has potent **antioxidant properties**. Unlike
other micronutrients, lycopene becomes **more available to the body after heating** and processing,
like in this tasty tomato sauce. And, as lycopene is
fat-soluble, consumption with **olive oil improves
absorption**.

ZUCCHINI FLOWERS AND SAFFRON RISOTTO

Total preparation time: **20 minutes**
Cooking time: **18 minutes**
Yield: **2 servings**

½ quart (about ½ liter) vegetable stock
½ pound (225 g) new zucchini (with flowers, if available)
3 tablespoons (about 40 g) unsalted butter
½ medium shallot, finely chopped
3/4 cup (about 140 g) Italian Carnaroli or Arborio rice
¼ cup (60 ml) dry white wine
¼ teaspoon saffron threads or 1/8 teaspoon saffron powder
⅓ cup (35 g) grated Parmesan cheese
Salt and freshly ground white pepper, to taste

1   In a saucepan over medium low heat, warm the stock.

2   Soak saffron threads or powder in 5 teaspoons of stock (warm, not boiling) for 15 minutes.

3   Cut flowers off from zucchini and remove pistil. Wash zucchini and flowers. Dice zucchini and slice flowers into thin strips.

4   In a large saucepan, heat 2 tablespoons butter. Add shallot and sauté for 2–3 minutes over medium heat. Add rice and stir thoroughly for about 3 minutes to coat the rice with butter and shallot. (This helps regulate the absorption of the liquid during cooking.) Add wine and stir until completely absorbed.

5   Add stock a soup ladle or two at a time until the rice is just covered and stir continuously with a wooden spoon. When

stock is almost completely absorbed, repeat this process for about 9 minutes.

6   Add diced zucchini and flowers and one more ladle of stock. Cook for another 5–6 minutes, until stock is nearly absorbed. Add prepared saffron. If you prefer softer zucchini, add diced zucchini at the beginning with the shallot.

7   **The end of the cooking is critical for the final texture of the dish.** When the rice is nearly tender but with just a hint of resistance (*al dente*) and the liquid you have added up to this point has been mostly absorbed (the *risotto* should still seem a bit "soupy"), remove *risotto* from heat. Add Parmesan cheese and the rest of the butter, to taste.

8   At this point, keep stirring the risotto to blend in the cheese and butter. You can also add some salt and freshly ground pepper, to taste. Let stand for 1–2 minutes. Arrange the risotto on a serving dish and serve immediately. Timing is everything; it is very easy to overcook risotto!

MAMMA MIA!

The addition of **saffron, the king of spices** (and the most expensive spice in the world by weight), makes your risotto dish something you will remember and want to make again and again. In addition to its culinary uses, **saffron** also has many **therapeutic properties** such as **anti-aging, anti-depressant, anti-cancer, and cardiovascular protection.**

Saffron adds an invitingly intense golden-yellow color (don't forget, we first eat with our eyes) and a special honey-like taste to this recipe. In fact, the word "saffron" originates from the Latin *safranum*, which in Arabic means yellow. Saffron comes from the stigmas of the flower *Crocus sativus* (commonly known as Saffron Crocus), cultivated in Asia Minor even before the birth of Christ and later brought into many Mediterranean countries. Egyptian physicians already cultivated this plant as early as 1,600 BCE. Today, the largest saffron crops in Italy are located in Abruzzo, Sardinia, Tuscany, and Umbria. The Aquila saffron (or *zafferano d'Aquila*), cultivated exclusively in the Navelli Valley, is among the best saffron in the world for its distinctive thread shape, unusually pungent aroma, and intense color.

Add saffron to your recipe and put some extra sunshine on your table—and into your life!

Zucchini flowers are available at many farmer's markets, but if you can't get a hold of them, regular zucchini works just as well!

DINNER

BAKED CHICKEN WITH HERBS AND BRUSSELS SPROUTS

Total preparation time: **30 minutes + 30 minutes marinating**
Cooking time: **30 minutes**
Yield: **2 servings**

Baked Chicken
½ free-range chicken (about 1 pound or 450 g) cut into four
    pieces
1 tablespoon dried hot chili pepper
1 tablespoon ground black pepper
1 garlic cloves, minced
½ tablespoon salt
½ tablespoon Dijon mustard
Juice of one organic lemon
1 sprig rosemary
1 sprig majoran
1 spring thyme
Brussels Sprouts
11 oz (310) Brussels sprouts, cleaned and washed
2 tablespoons extra virgin olive oil
2 tablespoons toasted almond flakes
Sea salt and freshly ground pepper, to taste

1   Wash chicken under running water and pat dry with paper
    towels.

2   Prepare marinade in a glass bowl by mixing dried hot chili
    pepper, pepper, garlic, salt, mustard, herbs, and lemon juice.
    You can increase the amount of spices according to your taste.

3   Add chicken and "massage" it by hand to coat well with spices.

4   Leave in the refrigerator for 30 minutes. If you do not have a lot of time, you can skip this step.

5   Preheat the oven to 400°F (200°C) and set oven rack to middle position.

6   In a large pan, add chicken with marinade. Cover with a lid and cook over medium-low heat for about 20–25 minutes until chicken is cooked thoroughly. Transfer chicken onto a baking sheet covered with parchment paper. Drizzle with some marinade and bake until golden brown.

7   While chicken is cooking, prepare Brussels sprouts. In a large pan, heat olive oil over medium heat. Add Brussels sprouts, season with salt and pepper, and cook, stirring frequently, until caramelized, about 8–10 minutes. Add ¼ cup water and cook until evaporated, about 2 minutes.

8   Sprinkle with toasted almonds and serve immediately with the chicken. Serve with a slice of whole grain bread, if desired.

MAMMA MIA!

Brussels sprouts fall into the cruciferous category of vegetables, which also includes broccoli and cabbage. This group of vegetables offers a unique composition of **antioxidants, vitamins (especially vitamins K and C), and minerals** that promote good health.

BAKED EGGPLANT ROLLS

Total preparation time: **20 minutes + 1 hour (for draining)**
Cooking time: **10 minutes**
Yield: **2 servings**

1 large eggplant (about 1 pound or 450 g)
1 scarce cup (about 220 ml) tomato sauce
½ pound (225 g) mozzarella for pizza, coarsely grated or
    seasoned ricotta cheese, crumbled
4 basil leaves + some for garnish
1 tablespoon extra-virgin olive oil + some for grilling
Kosher salt, to taste
Oregano and freshly ground pepper, to taste

1   Wash eggplant under cold water. Cut off ends and slice ver-
    tically into thin (¼ inch or 6 mm) slices. Arrange one layer
    of slices in the bottom of a large colander and sprinkle with
    kosher salt. Repeat this procedure until all eggplant slices are
    in the colander.

2   Weigh down slices with something heavy (for example, a few
    plates) and let them drain for at least one hour. This step helps
    release some of the bitter liquid before cooking.

3   In a saucepan over a medium-high heat, add 1 tablespoon of
    olive oil and the tomato sauce, a pinch of oregano, basil, and
    freshly ground pepper to taste. Cook over medium heat for
    2–3 minutes and set aside. I recommend using a dense tomato
    sauce rather than a liquid one.

4   Preheat the oven to 350°F (180°C) and set oven rack to middle
    position.

5   When eggplant slices have drained, press down on the slices to remove the excess water, wipe off the excess salt, and dry with paper towels.

6   Grill eggplant slices on a heated griddle lightly greased with some olive oil, turning once.

7   On each eggplant slice, spread half of a spoon of tomato sauce, cover with some mozzarella, and roll. (For the smaller slices, combine two lengthwise to have all the same length.) Repeat until all ingredients are used.

8   Place rolls either in two individual, lightly oiled baking pans or one larger one. Pour a teaspoon of tomato sauce on top of each roll and bake for 5–7 minutes, until mozzarella melts. Remove from oven and let rest on a grid for 2 minutes. Serve warm. You can enjoy this dish with steamed brown rice (1 serving is equal to ½ scarce cup or 70 g).

MAMMA MIA!

This is a quick, easy, and light way to prepare a delicious dish with eggplant (or *aubergine*, in French), a staple vegetable of Italian cuisine. **Eggplant** originates from Asia and gets its name from the first eggplants imported to America, which were round with a yellowish-white color (like an egg). The Italian name, "*melanzana*," means "*mela insana*" (or "insanity-apple") because when it was first introduced in Italy (around 1,500 CE), people thought the vegetable was noxious and could cause mental and intestinal disorders. Quite the contrary; in addition to being delicious, eggplant is very healthy. It is a good source of potassium, some fiber, and phytonutrients such as **anthocyanins** with **high antioxidant properties**. To retain these benefits, never peel an eggplant and buy organic ones where possible.

BAKED VEGETABLE FRITTATA

Total preparation time: **30 minutes**
Baking time: **15–20 minutes**
Yield: **4 servings**

2 medium potatoes (Yukon Gold), steamed and diced
2 medium carrots, peeled and cut into cubes
7–8 asparagus spears, cut into small pieces
1 cup (150 g) frozen peas
2 garlic cloves
4 tablespoons extra virgin olive oil
50 g (½ cup) grated Parmesan cheese
6 medium eggs (separate egg yolks from egg whites)
Sea salt and freshly ground pepper, to taste

1   Prepare a baking dish with parchment paper. Cut paper to be bigger than the baking dish, wash under running water, and wring the water out. Place paper in a ceramic or glass-baking dish (10 inches or 25 cm). Let edges go partially up the side of the dish to keep any batter from slipping into the baking dish. This method allows for a better adhesion of the paper to the dish wall. You can apply this method to any baking recipe.

2   Preheat the oven to 350°F (180°C) and set oven rack to middle position.

3   Wash potatoes under cold water. Peel and cut into 1 inch cubes (about 1 inch or 2.5 cm). Steam for about 6–8 minutes, until the potatoes are done but not soft. Set aside.

4   While potatoes are cooling, wash asparagus under cold water and trim the ends. Try to bend the stem; you will notice that at a certain point it will not bend, and that's the point where the stem begins to be tough.

5   In a large saucepan over medium heat, sauté garlic in olive oil until lightly browned. Remove it and add carrots, cook for a few minutes, then add asparagus. Cook until tender but still crisp. Stir in peas and cook for a few minutes. Add potatoes, mix gently, and set aside.

6   In a large bowl, beat egg yolks and add vegetable mixture, Parmesan cheese, salt, and pepper.

7   In a medium bowl, beat egg whites until fluffy. Combine egg whites with vegetable mix and pour into prepared baking dish.

8   Bake for about 15–20 minutes, or until custard is set and golden on top.

9   Remove from oven and allow to cool on a rack for about 7–8 minutes. Serve warm with a tasty salad. You can enjoy the *frittata* cold, too, and it is makes for a delicious lunch box dish.

MAMMA MIA!

Frittata is an **Italian-style omelet** made with beaten eggs and milk and enriched with various ingredients such as vegetables, cheese, ham, pasta, and herbs. There is technically a difference between a *frittata* and an omelet: an omelet's ingredients are placed on the omelet while it is cooking, while a *frittata* requires you to mix the eggs and other ingredients together before cooking.

You may have heard the expression **"hai fatto una frittata,"** which means (perhaps understandably) **"you made a mess**!" This expression comes from the fact that a *frittata* is usually made at the last minute with the ingredients available in the fridge—which includes leftovers! Good results are not always guaranteed.

Frittata is usually fried in a frying pan on the stove, but I prefer the **baking method** because it makes the *frittata* **healthier.**

BARLEY WITH PUMPKIN AND ALMONDS

Total preparation time: **45 minutes**
Cooking time: **40 minutes**
Yield: **2 servings**

¾ cup (150 g) barley
9 oz (250 g) pumpkin of *Mantua* (Cucurbita maxima, Kabocha)
    or butternut squash, peeled and diced)
½ medium shallot, finely chopped
2 tablespoons extra virgin olive oil
2 cups (about ½ liter) vegetable stock
1 sprig sage
2 tablespoons grated Parmesan cheese
2 tablespoons toasted almonds slices
Sea salt and freshly ground pepper, to taste

1   In a saucepan over medium heat, warm the stock. Wash barley
    under cold running water.

2   In a large saucepan over medium-low heat, sauté shallot in
    olive oil for 2–3 minutes until translucent and soft, but not
    browned. Add pumpkin and cook for 1 minute, stirring 2–3
    times. Add barley and stir thoroughly for about 2 minutes to
    coat the barley well with olive oil, shallot, and pumpkin.

3   Add a soup ladle or two of stock until barley is just covered,
    stirring continuously with a wooden spoon. When the stock is
    almost completely absorbed, add sage and repeat this process
    for about 35 minutes (depending on the barley's cooking time,
    which should be clearly indicated on the package).

4   Remove from heat. Add Parmesan cheese, pepper, and salt,
     if necessary (depending on the amount of salt present in the
     stock). Before serving, top with almonds. Serve immediately.

MAMMA MIA!

Pumpkin is an autumn vegetable. In addition to being a tasty ingredient in many recipes, it is a very healthy choice, as it is an **excellent source of beta-carotene (pro-vitamin A) and minerals (calcium and phosphorus) and a good source of fiber.** Pumpkin is low in calories and contains lots of water, making it a perfect ingredient to use in a **weight loss plan.**

BEEF FILLET WITH MUSHROOMS

Total preparation time: **50 minutes**
Baking time: **30 minutes**
Yield: **3–4 servings**

Porcini mushrooms
½ pound (225 g) *Porcini* mushrooms or champignons
    mushrooms
1–2 garlic cloves, minced
1 tablespoon parsley, finely chopped
1½ tablespoons extra virgin olive oil
Roast Fillet
13 oz (360 g) beef fillet or tenderloin roast
Balsamic vinegar
1–2 garlic cloves
2 tablespoons extra virgin olive oil
1 sprig rosemary
1 sprig sage
Sea salt and freshly ground pepper, to taste

1   Preheat the oven to 475°F (250°C) and set oven rack to middle
    position.

2   To clean the mushrooms, wipe them off with a moist cloth.
    Use a knife, if necessary, to remove any remaining soil. Slice
    the mushrooms vertically into ⅛ inch (3 mm) strips. Many
    say not to wash *porcini* mushrooms with water, but I prefer
    to do so. If you wash them, do it immediately before slicing
    and cooking, and dry immediately with some paper towels.
    When cooking, it is important to use either a nonstick or a
    steel pan, because other metals in contact with the *porcini* can
    release toxic compounds. *Porcini* are well suited to drying, and
    actually, the flavor of dried mushrooms is more intense. Before

using dried mushrooms, soak them in hot, but not boiling, water for about twenty minutes.

3   In a large saucepan over medium-high heat, sauté garlic in olive oil until lightly browned. Remove it. Stir in mushrooms, salt to taste, and cook for approximately 7 minutes. Continue to cook for 1–2 minutes over high heat. Add parsley and set aside.

4   Before cooking fillet, season with salt and pepper and let stand unrefrigerated until it reaches room temperature, about 20 minutes. You can also marinate the garlic with olive oil for at least two hours.

5   In a large roasting pan, rub olive oil seasoned with garlic all over the meat. Lay rosemary and sage sprigs in the bottom of the roasting pan and place fillet roast on top of them. Sprinkle balsamic vinegar on the meat.

6   Place roast in the oven for about 8–10 minutes. Reduce heat to 350°F (180°C) and cook for additional 15–18 minutes. Use a meat thermometer to determine when it reaches your preferred level of doneness (125°F/50°C for rare and 135°/55°C for medium-rare).

7   Remove roast from the oven and let stand covered with aluminum foil for about 10 minutes before serving.

8   Heat mushrooms and serve on top of the meat. You can also enjoy this dish with some steamed potatoes (1 serving is equal to 1 medium potato) or steamed broccoli.

MAMMA MIA!

The Italian name *porcini* (pronounced *"por-CHEE-nee"*) means "piglets," probably owing to the fondness pigs have for eating them! **Porcini** have **more protein** than most other vegetables apart from legumes and soybeans. They also contain some **vitamins (such as niacin), minerals (potassium, phosphorus), and fiber. They have no fat and only a few calories.** *Porcini* have a nutty and slightly meaty taste with a smooth and creamy texture. Young, small *porcini* are tastier than older and larger ones.

CHICKEN BREAST WITH PEPPERS

Total preparation time: **25 minutes**
Cooking time: **15 minutes**
Yield: **2 servings**

10 oz (280 g) chicken breast
3 tablespoons extra virgin olive oil
1 sprig fresh rosemary
1 hot dried chili pepper
1/2 cup (120 ml) dry white wine
7 oz (200 g) canned tomatoes (San Marzano)
1 garlic clove
2 medium bell peppers of different colors
1/2 teaspoon sugar
Sea salt and freshly ground black pepper, to taste

1   In a saucepan, heat 2 tablespoons of olive oil, then sauté
    chicken on medium heat for a few minutes until golden brown
    on both sides.

2   Add rosemary and chili pepper. Season with salt and freshly
    ground pepper. Add white wine and cook for about 8–10
    minutes (the meat should be tender).

3   While chicken is cooking, prepare peppers. Wash and cut
    in half, removing seeds and white filaments. Cut into pieces
    about 1.5 in (3 cm) in width.

4   In a nonstick pan over medium-low heat, sauté a garlic clove
    in 1 tablespoon of olive oil until lightly browned, then remove.
    Add peppers, increasing the heat to medium, and cook for 5
    minutes, stirring frequently. Add tomatoes and salt. Cook with
    the lid on for about 10–15 minutes, until the peppers are soft.

5   Serve peppers on top of chicken. You can enjoy with some
     steamed rice (1 serving is equal to 1/4 cup or 45 g).

MAMMA MIA!

This is a tasty Roman dish that can be prepared with a whole chicken cut into six pieces, as well. The combination of peppers and the delicate **lean chicken meat** creates a truly inviting and healthy dish. The addition of chili pepper gives a special bite to this recipe. The amount of chili pepper is purely personal; if you want a really spicy dish, you can always add more!

SCALLOPS AU GRATIN

Total preparation time: **15 minutes**
Baking time: **10 minutes**
Yield: **2 servings**

8 bay scallops
3.5 oz (100 g) bread crumbs
2 tablespoons extra virgin olive oil
1 sprig thyme
1 sprig majoran
1 sprig parsley
1 garlic clove, minced
Zest of 1 organic lemon
Sea salt and freshly ground pepper, to taste

1   Preheat the oven to 400°F (200°C) and set oven rack to t
    middle position.

2   Wash scallops under cold running water and pat dry with
    paper towel.

3   Process bread crumbs, olive oil, thyme, majoran, parsley, gar-
    lic, lemon zest, salt, and pepper in a blender or food processor.

4   Place scallops in a shallow baking pan and sprinkle with the
    bread crumbs mix.

5   Bake for 10 minutes until golden. Remove and serve
    immediately.

MAMMA MIA!

In addition to their delectable taste, scallops are a shell-fish which contain a variety of nutrients that can promote your cardiovascular health and prevent colon cancer. Scallops are also an excellent source of vitamin B12, potassium, magnesium, and selenium, and are low in saturated fat.

VEGGIE-BALLS

Total preparation time: **45 minutes**
Cooking time: **20 minutes**
Yield: **4 servings**

1 medium onion, finely diced
2 garlic cloves
2 medium carrots, finely diced
1 medium red bell pepper, finely diced
2 zucchini, finely diced
1¾ cups (250 g) frozen peas
¼ cup (60 ml) extra virgin olive oil + some for baking
5 oz (140 g) creamy ricotta cheese
½ cup (about 50 g) grated Parmesan cheese
1 medium size egg
4–5 tablespoons bread crumbs + extra for rolling
Sea salt, freshly ground pepper and grated nutmeg, to taste
Fresh parsley or mint leaves, to taste

1   Preheat the oven to 400°F (200°F) and set oven rack to middle position.

2   In nonstick pan, sauté onion and garlic in olive oil over medium heat for 4 minutes, stirring frequently. Remove garlic.

3   Add carrots and bell pepper, tossing for a few minutes.

4   Add zucchini and cook for 7 minutes.

5   Add peas and cook for an additional 4–5 minutes, stirring a few times to prevent burning. Add salt and pepper, to taste. Set aside and let cool.

6   In a bowl, mix ricotta cheese with Parmesan and egg. Add vegetable mix and 4–5 tablespoons of bread crumbs. The resulting

dough shouldn't be too wet. Adjust salt and add nutmeg to taste. You can add some fresh parsley leaves or some mint (finely chopped), as well. Place dough in the refrigerator for 20 minutes.

7   Place some parchment paper on a baking sheet. Lightly sprinkle with some olive oil.

8   Roll about 1 tablespoon of dough into a ball. Roll in the bread crumbs and then place on the baking sheet, turning once to lightly coat with some olive oil all around. Repeat until all dough is used.

9   Bake for 7–8 minutes, turning at least once, until light golden browned. Remove from oven, let cool for a few minutes, and serve warm. (But they're good cold, too—a perfect lunch box food!)

MAMMA MIA!

Fresh vegetables make these "veggie-balls" a perfect and colorful dish for **vegetarians**, but they're also tasty enough also for the "carnivores" at your table, too.

I prefer **baking** them rather as opposed to frying, because you need less fat and the result is *obviously* **healthier**.

BEETS AND RICOTTA DUMPLINGS

Total preparation time: **30 minutes**
Total cooking time: **8–10 minutes**
Yield: **2 servings**

¾ cup (135 g) cooked, peeled and diced beets
½ heaping cup (150 g) cow's or goat's milk strained ricotta
cheese
⅓ heaping cup (about 40 g) grated Parmesan cheese
¾ cup (100 g) all-purpose flour
1 pinch grated nutmeg
2 tablespoons unsalted butter
4 sage leaves, cut into large pieces
2 tablespoons grated Parmesan cheese
Sea salt and freshly ground pepper, to taste

1   Process beets in a blender until smooth. Add ricotta and blend until ingredients are just mixed.

2   Transfer the beet dough into a bowl. Add Parmesan and season with nutmeg and fresh ground pepper. Mix with a spoon and let rest in the refrigerator for 15 minutes.

3   Bring a large pot of salted water to boil (about 1 scarce teaspoon of sea salt per 1 quart or 1 liter of water).

4   Remove beets from refrigerator and add flour. Mix gently until completely incorporated. Be careful not to overwork it; the dough should be light and the texture soft.

5   Drop teaspoon-sized balls of dough (using another spoon to
      scrape out the dough) into the boiling water. Before cooking
      the whole batch, I recommend making a couple test dump-
      lings to see if dough holds together. Cooked *gnocchi* (dump-
      lings) should be firm but not tough, and should not fall apart
      in the water. If they fall apart, add 1–2 tablespoons of flour. If
      they are tough, then you've used too much flour.

6   In a saucepan melt butter and add sage leaves. Cook over
      medium heat to flavor butter.

7   Cook *gnocchi* for about 45–50 seconds after they float to the
      top. Remove with a slotted spoon or spider spoon and place in
      the saucepan. Repeat with the remaining dough and toss gen-
      tly. You can serve with some pepper and grated Parmesan. As
      a starter, enjoy a green salad with tomatoes, olives, and boiled
      eggs (1 serving is equal to 1–2 medium eggs).

MAMMA MIA!

Gnocchi (pronounced gnawk-KEY) or dumplings with beets and ricotta, is a classic winter dish when beets are in season in Italy. *Gnocchi* is an easy, fast, and light recipe to prepare, although you do need to take care in minimizing the amount of flour used. I grew up making *gnocchi al cucchiaio*—gnocchi made with a spoon, a typical Lombard recipe—with my mom, especially on Fridays. In fact, *gnocchi* is considered a weekday dish.

Beets have an intense color due to pigments **called betalains**, which give them an impressive, inviting look in addition to their **healthy benefits. Beets are not only beautiful, but are also a unique source of phytonutrients that have been shown to provide antioxidant, anti-inflammatory, and detoxifying properties.** Betalains are steadily released from food as cooking time is increased, so I recommend that you keep steaming times for beets to 15 minutes or less, and roasting times to under an hour. For this reason, I also suggest purchasing small or medium-sized beets. Smaller, younger beets are tenderer and cook faster. In Italy, you can purchase pre-steamed or roasted beets from the local supermarket, meaning you don't need to cook them yourself.

CODFISH WITH GINGER AND PINE NUTS

Total preparation time: **20 minutes + 30 minutes marinating**
Baking time: **20 minutes**
Yield: **2 servings**

11 oz (310 g) codfish fillets
2 tablespoons extra virgin olive oil
½ organic lemon, juice
½ small chili pepper, finely sliced without seeds
½ inch (about 1 cm) fresh ginger roof, peeled and grated
1–2 garlic cloves, minced
10 oz (280 g) cherry tomatoes
2 tablespoons pine nuts, toasted
2 tablespoons black olives
Fresh thyme, to taste
Sea salt and freshly ground pepper, to taste

1   Wash fish fillets under cold running water and pat dry with
     paper towels.

2   Prepare marinade by mixing the olive oil, lemon juice, chili
     pepper, ginger, and garlic together in a bowl.

3   Place fillets in a glass *container* and pour the marinade *over*
     it. Cover with plastic wrap and let rest in the refrigerator for
     20–30 minutes.

4   Preheat the oven to 375°F (200°C) and set oven rack to middle
     position. Place some parchment paper on a shallow baking
     dish.

5 Add marinade, tomatoes, and olives to the baking dish. Season with salt and pepper. Remove the fillets from the refrigerator and let it sit at room temperature for 8 minutes.

6 Bake for 10–12 minutes. Add cod fillets amongst the vegetables, adding pine nuts on top, and cooking for an additional 8–10 minutes (depending on the size of the fillets).

7 Remove from oven, sprinkle some fresh thyme, and serve warm. You can enjoy with some steamed basmati rice (1 serving is equal to about ¼ cup or 45 g).

MAMMA MIA!

Codfish has a mild flavor and a dense, flaky white flesh. Codfish is **rich in protein** and has a **high mineral** content consisting mainly of phosphorus and potassium.

CRISP SEA BASS WITH ASPARAGUS

Total preparation time: **20 minutes**
Cooking time: **15 minutes**
Yield: **2 servings**

2 sea bass filets (about 10 oz or 280 g skin-on, scaled, scored,
    and pin-boned)
3 tablespoons extra virgin olive oil
Zest of 1 organic lemon
1 organic lemon, cut into wedges
Fresh ginger root (½ inch or about 1 cm), peeled and grated
1 pound (450 g) asparagus
¼ cup (60 ml) vegetable broth
½ cup (75 g) frozen peas
2 tablespoons toasted almonds slices
Salt and pepper, to taste

1   Prepare vegetables. Wash asparagus under cold running water.
     Trim the ends. Try to bend the stem; you will notice that at
     certain point it will not break, which is the point where the
     stem begins to be tough. Scrape the length of the stem with
     a knife, taking care not to break the tips. Rinse again under
     running cold water and cut into pieces about ½ an inch (1.25
     cm) long, while keeping the top intact.

2   In a pan, sauté asparagus in 2 tablespoons olive oil over
     medium heat for about 2–3 minutes. Season with salt and add
     broth. Add peas and cook, covered, for about 5–10 minutes
     on low heat (depending on the size of the asparagus and the
     tenderness of the peas). When done, remove the lid and turn
     up the heat to let the remaining liquid evaporate.

3 While vegetables are cooking, wash filets under cold running water and pat dry with some paper towels. Sprinkle the skin of the fish with salt and rub all over with the remaining olive oil.

4 Heat a heavy-based griddle until very hot (this can take up to 8–10 minutes). Add filets (skin side down) and season with salt, lemon zest, and pepper. Cook for 4–5 minutes until crisp.

5 Top vegetables with almonds, add some pepper, and stir to mix the flavors.

6 Turn the griddle heat to medium-high. Turn filets with a spatula and continue cooking until just done and crisp on top, about 3–4 minutes (depending on the thickness of filet). Serve immediately with the asparagus and lemon wedges for squeezing over the fish.

MAMMA MIA!

Whether you eat **sea or freshwater bass,** the bottom line is it's healthy for you. **Low in calories** and an **excellent source of protein, minerals** (potassium, phosphorus), and **vitamins** (especially vitamin A), bass is **low in total fat,** with both varieties being good **sources of two omega-3 fatty acids:** EPA and DHA.

GNUDI (SPINACH AND RICOTTA DUMPLINGS)

Total preparation time: **35–40 minutes**
Cooking time: **10 minutes**
Yield: **2 servings**

12.5 oz (350 g) fresh spinach leaves
1 scarce cup (210 g) strained sheep or cow's milk ricotta
½ cup (70 g) all-purpose flour + some extra for rolling the
    dough
½ tablespoon extra-virgin olive oil
1 garlic clove
1 small egg
¼ cup (30 g) grated Parmesan cheese
1 pinch nutmeg
2 tablespoons unsalted butter
1 sprig sage
2 tablespoons grated Parmesan cheese
Sea salt and freshly ground pepper, to taste

1   Wash spinach under running cold water and steam for a few
    minutes. Transfer to a colander placed over a bowl to drain
    excess fluid, crushing with a spoon or squeezing with your
    hands to facilitate excess water release.

2   In a large saucepan, heat olive oil over medium heat and sauté
    garlic until lightly browned. Remove garlic and stir in spinach,
    cooking for a few minutes. Let cool completely. If there is
    excess water, drain again. Finely chop with a knife.

3   Bring a large pot of salted water to boil (about 1 scarce tea-
    spoon of sea salt per 1 quart or liter of water).

4   Pour ricotta and spinach (well drained) into a large bowl. Sea-
    son with nutmeg, salt and pepper. Add egg, Parmesan cheese,
    and flour. Mix well to obtain a firm dough.

5   Roll about one tablespoon of dough into a ball in the flour
    and place on a baking sheet covered with parchment paper.
    Continue until you finish all the dough.

6   Drop each dumpling into the boiling water, cooking for about
    35–40 seconds after they float to the top. Place *gnocchi* on a
    warm plate and serve with melted butter with sage and Parme-
    san cheese.

MAMMA MIA!

Like most dishes, **gnocchi** are better consumed fresh
and right away. Homemade tomato sauce with fresh
basil is an alternative seasoning to butter and sage.

GRILLED SALMON STEAK WITH SPINACH

Total preparation time: **10 minutes + 45–50 minutes marinating**
Cooking time: **6–8 minutes**
Yield: **2 servings**

Salmon
2 middle-cut boneless salmon filets (12.5 oz or 350 g)
3 tablespoons extra virgin olive oil
Juice of 1 medium size organic lemon
1 lemon (for garnishing)
2 sprigs dill
Sea salt and freshly ground pepper, to taste
Spinach
2 pounds (900 g) fresh spinach leaves
2 tablespoons extra virgin olive oil
2 garlic cloves
Sea salt and freshly ground pepper, to taste

1   In a small bowl, combine olive oil, lemon juice, dill, and pepper.

2   Wash salmon filets under cold running water and pat dry with some paper towels.

3   Place filets in a shallow pan. Add marinade and cover with plastic wrap. Refrigerate for 45–50 minutes.

4   Remove filets from the refrigerator and let them sit at room temperature while you pre-heat the griddle.

5   Heat a heavy-based griddle until very hot (this can take up to 8–10 minutes). Add salmon, seasoning with salt (additional) and pepper.

6   Cook for 3–4 minutes; by this time, a good crust should have formed. Turn with a spatula and continue cooking until just done, about 3–4 minutes, depending on the thickness of the filet. The salmon should be just cooked through when done.

7   While salmon is cooking, prepare spinach. Wash spinach under running cold water. Place in a large saucepan and cook, covered, over medium heat for 4–5 minutes. Spinach should be tender but not mushy.

8   Transfer to a bowl with cold water and ice and let rest for 1–2 minutes. Drain in a colander placed over a bowl. To remove the excess water, crush with a spoon or squeeze with your hands.

9   In a large saucepan, heat olive oil over medium heat and sauté garlic until lightly browned. Remove garlic and stir in spinach, seasoning with salt and pepper. Cook for a few minutes, stirring occasionally.

10 1Serve salmon with spinach and a thin slice of lemon. Enjoy with some steamed basmati rice (1 serving is equal to about ¼ cup or 45 g).

MAMMA MIA!

Salmon is an excellent source of **high-quality protein, some vitamins (A and B3), minerals** (especially potassium and phosphorus), and **omega-3 fatty acids**, which should receive special attention. If you like, you can enrich this recipe by adding a tablespoon of roasted pine nuts to spinach before serving.

GRILLED TUNA STEAK

Total preparation time: **15 minutes**
Cooking time: **4–5 minutes**
Yield: **2 servings**

12.5 oz (350 g) fresh tuna steak
2 tablespoons poppy seeds or sesame seeds
1 tablespoon extra-virgin olive oil
Sea salt and freshly ground pepper, to taste
Balsamic vinegar glaze

1   Rinse tuna steak with cold running water and pat dry with paper towels.

2   Grease a grill with some olive oil. Preheat the grill to medium.

3   Brush tuna steak with the olive oil and encrust with poppy seeds.

4   Grill for about 4 minutes for each ½ inch (1.25 cm) thickness, turning once halfway through to promote even cooking. The center of the steak should be pink, so it remains tender and moist.

5   Cut steak into ½ inch (1.25 cm) slices and season with salt, pepper and balsamic vinegar glaze. Serve immediately with grilled vegetables and sliced rustic Italian bread (1 serving is equal to 1 slice).

MAMMA MIA!

Tuna fish of varying species and sizes are found in all of the world's oceans. Tuna is a **great source of omega-3 fatty acids,** an excellent **source of protein** (22% in 3.5 oz or 100 g), **selenium, and some vitamins (B3 and A), and low in cholesterol.**

When buying tuna steak, be certain that it is fresh and from small fish. Mercury content increases in larger fish, so it is better to avoid the larger species like albacore. Cook fish the same day you purchase it. If frozen, thaw in the refrigerator for at least one day.

HUNTER'S CHICKEN STEW

Total preparation time: **1 hour 10 minutes**
Cooking time: **55 minutes**
Yield: **4 servings**

2¼ pounds (about 1 kg) chicken (or rabbit), cut into six pieces
4 tablespoons extra virgin olive oil
1 sprig fresh rosemary
2 garlic cloves, finely chopped
2 medium carrots, finely sliced
1 medium onion, finely sliced
2 celery stalks, finely sliced
5 sage leaves
240 ml (1 cup) dry white wine
1 pound (450 g) canned tomatoes (such as *S. Marzano*)
½ pound (225 g) champignons mushrooms, cleaned and thickly
    sliced
½ cup (120 ml) vegetable stock (optional)
½–1 tablespoon parsley, finely chopped
Sea salt and freshly ground black pepper, to taste

1   Heat olive oil in a large nonstick pan, and cook chicken over
    medium-high heat for about 10 minutes, until golden brown
    on both sides.

2   Add rosemary, sage, and vegetables. Season with salt and
    freshly ground pepper, to taste. Cook for 4–5 minutes. Add
    wine and let it simmer until half of it has evaporated.

3   Add tomatoes. Cover and cook for about 20 minutes. Remove
    the lid and add mushrooms. Cook for an additional 15–20
    minutes until the flesh is tender, stirring occasionally. If liquid
    evaporates, add some vegetable stock.

4   Add a little salt and pepper to taste, if desired. Remove rose-
     mary sprig, sprinkle parsley on top, and serve immediately
     with steamed broccoli.

MAMMA MIA!

A typical peasant dish, **coniglio alla cacciatora** is an
appetizing main course. While we've presented it here
using chicken, for a truly authentic Italian experience you
must try it using rabbit, which is most commonly available at farmer's markets. If using rabbit, prepare it by
cutting the rabbit into pieces, removing the head and
entrails. To save time, ask the butcher to clean it properly
it for you. Wash and dry with paper towels. If you clean
the rabbit yourself, soak for 2–3 hours in cold water with
lemon juice to eliminate the gamey taste. Wash and dry
with paper towels.

Did you know that the rabbit is actually native to
Africa? It was later imported to Europe, especially
to Italy and France. The Italian name *coniglio* derives
from the Latin word *cuniculus*, referring to the ability of
this animal to dig warrens with many tunnels (*cunicoli*).
Rabbit is a **lean meat**, making it a healthy choice as
compared to beef and pork.

MARINATED CHICKEN BREAST IN ORANGE JUICE WITH PISTACHIOS

Total preparation time: **15 minutes + 30 minutes marinating**
Cooking time: **10 minutes**
Yield: **2 servings**

10 oz (280 g) chicken breast, sliced and pounded
2 medium blood or Navel oranges + 1 orange, finely sliced, for
   garnish
2 tablespoons toasted granola pistachios + some whole
   pistachios for garnish
Salt and freshly ground pepper, to taste

1   In a nonstick pan, toast granola pistachios over medium heat.
    Stir often, making sure not to let it burn. Cool and set aside.

2   Squeeze orange and place chicken in a glass container. Pour on
    orange juice, cover with plastic wrap, and store in the refriger-
    ator for 30 minutes.

3   Heat a nonstick pan to medium. Pour in chicken with orange
    juice and cook until juice glazes. While cooking, add salt and
    pepper to taste.

4   Decorate a serving plate with orange slices, arrange chicken as
    desired, and add granola pistachios on top (with some whole
    pistachios, too). Serve warm with steamed basmati rice (1
    serving is equal to about ¼ cup or 45 g) and sautéed vegetables
    on the side.

MAMMA MIA!

In just this one recipe, you can combine all the health benefits of a wide variety of foods. **Chicken breast** is a very **lean meat, rich in protein,** that helps you get the best fitness and sports results. **Oranges** are loaded with **vitamin C, a potent antioxidant which helps control inflammatory diseases.** It's also packed with **pectin, which has been linked to cholesterol and diabetes control. Sicilian blood oranges** contain antioxidant red compounds—**anthocyanins**—which are present in many fruits, but which are uncommon in citrus fruit, making these oranges very special! **Pistachios** are a good source of main nutrients (for more information, refer to page 44). In just one recipe, you can combine all the health benefits of a wide variety of foods.

MONKFISH WITH CHERRY TOMATOES AND OLIVES

Total preparation time: **30 minutes**
Baking time: **20 minutes**
Yield: **2 servings**

12 oz (340 g) monkfish medallions
½ pound (225 g) cherry tomatoes
1 garlic clove, crushed
1½ tablespoons bread crumbs
1 tablespoon dried oregano
2 tablespoons black olives or Italian Taggiasche olives, pitted
Extra virgin olive oil
Sea salt and freshly ground pepper, to taste

1   Preheat the oven to 350°F (180°C) and set oven rack to middle position.

2   Wash tomatoes and cut into quarters. Place in a bowl and dress with 1 tablespoon olive oil, garlic, oregano, and a pinch of salt and pepper. Remove ½ of the liquid.

3   Wash fish under running water (not for too long, as its meat is particularly delicate) and pat dry with paper towels.

4   Drizzle a ceramic baking pan with some olive oil. Place fish in it, and top with tomato mix, olives, and bread crumbs.

5   Bake for about 15–20 minutes. Serve warm with steamed potatoes (1 serving is equal to 1 medium potato).

MAMMA MIA!

Monkfish is also known as angler fish (when it is cleaned, headless, and ready for cooking, is called monkfish; otherwise, it's an angler fish). At the fish market or supermarket, you will rarely find it with the head for one simple reason: it is not a particularly beautiful fish to look at, and for this reason the head is removed. Despite its ugly looks, angler fish has very tasty and lean meat. It is **low in calories** and rich in a lot of nutrients: **vitamins** (B3 and B12), **minerals** (selenium, potassium and phosphorus), omega-3 fatty acids, and **high-quality protein.**

RED LENTIL PUREE WITH GRILLED PRAWNS

Total preparation time: **30 minutes + soaking time**
Cooking time: **20 minutes**
Yield: **2 servings**

Lentils
1 scarce cup (170 g) red lentils
½ medium onion, finely chopped
1 garlic clove, finely chopped
½ medium carrot, finely diced
½ celery stem, finely diced
2 bay leaves
3 tablespoons extra virgin olive oil
60 ml (¼ cup) champagne or dry white wine
Vegetable stock
½ inch (about 1 cm) ginger root, peeled and grated
Sea salt and freshly ground pepper, to taste
Prawns
12 prawns, shelled and deveined
2 tablespoons extra virgin olive oil
1 garlic clove

1   In a large bowl, soak lentils for at least 2–3 hours, changing water once or twice. If you don't have time, you can also cook lentils straight away without soaking.

2   In a saucepan over medium heat, add olive oil, then onion, garlic, carrot, and celery and sauté over medium-low for a few minutes, stirring a few times with a wooden spoon.

3   Rinse lentils under running water and add lentils to saucepan.
    Cook on high heat for a few minutes, stirring with a wooden
    spoon.

4   Add wine and let it evaporate. Add bay leaves and cover with
    plenty of stock. Cover with a lid and cook over medium-low
    for about 18–20 minutes, until lentils are tender (the exact
    cooking time will be indicated on the package). Add salt and
    freshly ground pepper to taste.

5   Remove from heat. Remove bay leaves and purée lentils with
    a blender (the purée should be very smooth). Test for taste,
    adjusting salt and pepper accordingly. Grate ginger and mix
    with a spoon to blend all flavors. Keep warm.

6   Wash prawns and pat dry with paper towels. In a nonstick
    saucepan, heat olive oil over medium heat. Add garlic and
    prawns. Adjust pepper and sauté for a few minutes until they
    turn just pinkish-red.

7   Place lentils on a serving plate and decorate with prawns.
    Serve immediately.

MAMMA MIA!

Lentils have been a staple in the human diet since
ancient times. Available in dozens of types, lentils vary
in color, size, and texture, but all have similar nutritional
values. For more information, refer to page 41.

RIBOLLITA SOUP

Total preparation time: **2 hours**
Cooking time: **1½ hour**
Yield: **4 servings**

2 garlic cloves, peeled and finely chopped + 1 whole clove (for
    the bread)
½ medium onion, peeled and finely chopped
1 large carrots, peeled and finely sliced
½ celery stalk, finely sliced
1 large potato, peeled and diced
2.5 oz (70 g) pumpkin, peeled, cleaned and diced
4.5 oz (125 g) white kidney beans, already cooked (see *Note*)
4.5 oz (125 g) cranberry beans, already cooked (see *Note*)
4.5 oz (125 g) kale leaves, finely sliced
3.5 oz (100 g) Savory cabbage leaves, finely sliced
3 Swiss chard leaves, finely sliced
1 medium size tomato, peeled and coarsely chopped or 2
    tablespoons tomato sauce
2 tablespoons extra virgin olive oil
Sea salt and freshly ground pepper, to taste
Tuscan bread
Grated pecorino cheese (optional)

1   In a large saucepan over medium-low heat, sauté garlic, onion,
    carrot, and celery in olive oil for a few minutes. Add pumpkin
    and potato. Cook for 1–2 minutes to mix flavors.

2   Add half of the beans and the rest of the vegetables. If using
    canned beans, rinse them several times under cold running
    water.

3   Add 2 cups (about ½ liter) of water and salt and pepper
     (according to taste) and cook covered with a lid for about 1½
     hours. Add rest of the beans 5 minutes before removing from
     heat.

4   Slice bread and toast it, either on a grill or under a broiler. Rub
     with a clove of garlic cut in half.

5   Place a slice of bread in a bowl, cover with soup, drizzle olive
     oil on top, and add freshly ground pepper to taste. Serve hot,
     topped with freshly grated pecorino cheese (though the tradi-
     tional recipe does not call for it). If you'd like to enjoy the real
     ribollita experience, prepare the soup the day before you plan
     to eat it. Re-heat it and enjoy!

MAMMA MIA!

The word *ribollita* means "boiled again" and refers to the
fact that it was prepared the day before and warmed up
before eating the next day.

Of course, throughout Tuscany (where *ribollita* comes
from) each province, city, and town has its own version,
meaning there is no standard recipe. Nonetheless, there
is a basic rule: to really be called *ribollita*, your vegetable soup must include beans and two kinds of cabbage:
Savory cabbage and kale.

For nutritional information about kale, refer to *Pasta
with Kale* on page 220.

Note: To prepare using dried beans, you should plan to start the day before preparing the soup. (Keep in mind that 3.5 oz (100 g) dried beans are equal to 8.5 oz (240 g) cooked beans.) Rinse the beans under running water, then place in a large glass bowl with two bay leaves. Fill the bowl with plenty of water, enough to cover the beans generously (about 2 inches or 5 cm above the level of the beans). Cover with a lid and soak overnight.

The next day, remove the water and bay leaves, rinse the beans, and cook in plenty of water on medium-low heat covered with a lid. Add salt only just before they are done.

SICILIAN FISH SALAD

Total preparation time: **30 minutes**
Cooking time: **10 minutes**
Yield: **2 servings**

12.5 oz (350 g) codfish, cleaned, washed and pat dried
1 celery stalk, cut in fine slices
7 oz (200 g) *Pachino* tomatoes or cherry tomatoes, cut in half
6–7 green olives, pitted and sliced
1 tablespoon capers under salt, washed and dried
2 medium small potatoes
2 tablespoons extra virgin olive oil
½ organic lemon, juice
Sea salt and freshly ground pepper, to taste

1   In a large pan filled with salted water, cook whole potatoes over medium heat for about 20–25 minutes. Cooking time will vary according to size. They should be tender but not crumbly. Drain and allow to cool, and then peel and cut each potato into 10–12 pieces.

2   Season fish with some lemon juice. Pour 3–4 inches (7–10 cm) of water into a pan. Make sure that a steamer can sit on top of the pan with some space between the water and the bottom level of the steamer. Turn heat to high and bring water to a boil. Place fish in the steamer, cover, and cook for 8–10 minutes. Cooking time will depend on the thickness of fish; a 1½ inch (about 4 cm) thick filet will take about 10 minutes. Take care not to overcook it.

3   Remove from heat and let cool completely in the water. Then, remove from pan and cut into pieces about 1½ inches (about 4 cm).

4   In a large bowl, mix celery, tomatoes, olives, capers, potatoes and parsley.

5   In a small bowl, prepare dressing by mixing olive oil, lemon juice, salt, and pepper.

6   Gently toss salad with dressing and add fish cut into pieces. Toss gently; you do not want to break the fish. Serve immediately, or cover with some plastic wrap and let rest in the refrigerator for 1 hour.

MAMMA MIA!

This is a tasty salad to enjoy on a hot summer *day* when tomatoes are in season. For more information on codfish, refer to *Codfish with Ginger and Pine Nuts* on page 258.

STUFFED PEPPERS

Preparation time: **50–55 minutes**
Baking time: **45–50 minutes**
Yield: **2–3 servings**

2 medium bell peppers of different colors and rounded shape
7 oz (200 g) minced beef
3.5 oz (100 g) minced chicken breast
¼ cup (60 ml) milk
1.5 oz (40 g) day-old bread, soaked in milk and squeezed
1 medium egg
¼ cup (about 30 g) grated Parmesan
1–2 cloves garlic, finely chopped
1 sprig parsley, finely chopped
Extra virgin olive oil
Salt and freshly ground pepper, to taste

1   Preheat oven to 400°F (200°C) and set oven rack to middle
    position.

2   Wash peppers under running water. *Using* a small knife, cut
    top off and set aside. Scoop out seeds and filaments. Rinse and
    dry. Make a small cut or hole on both sides of each pepper
    using the point of a knife.

3   Wash and dry parsley. Peel garlic and chop finely with parsley.

4   In a bowl, mix meats, bread crumbs, egg, Parmesan, chopped
    parsley and garlic, salt, and freshly ground pepper.

5   Stuff peppers with the mixture. Cover with the tops and place
    peppers in an ovenproof dish. Drizzle a little oil on top of
    each pepper and cook for about 30 minutes, covered with
    aluminum foil. Remove foil and continue cooking for another

15 minutes. Peppers should be golden and tender. Serve warm with steamed basmati rice (1 serving is equal to about ¼ cup or 45 g).

MAMMA MIA!

Peppers, despite being from South America, were imported to continental Europe and cultivated in the Mediterranean area. They have been part of our Italian cuisine for many centuries. Peppers are vegetables **rich in vitamin A and C, beta-carotene,** and **minerals** (mainly potassium).

ZUCCHINI SPAGHETTI WITH PESTO AND CHERRY TOMATOES

Preparation time: **10 minutes**
Yield: **2 servings**

3 medium zucchini
3 tablespoons fresh pesto
5 cherry tomatoes, cut into small pieces
5 oz (140 g) or about 2 slices of sheep or cow's milk ricotta
    cheese
Salt (optional)
Freshly ground pepper, to taste
2 tablespoons toasted pine nuts (for garnish)

1   Wash zucchini. Cut off ends and cut into julienne spaghetti-strips using a spiral vegetable cutter.

2   In a bowl, season the zucchini spaghetti with two tablespoons of pesto and cherry tomatoes. Add salt (optional, because pesto is salty) and pepper to taste.

3   Arrange spaghetti on a serving dish and garnish with ricotta slices, remaining pesto, and some pine nuts. Serve immediately with sliced rustic bread (1 scrving is equal to 1 slice).

MAMMA MIA!

Turn your zucchini into pasta! In just a few minutes, you can prepare a large quantity of *spaghetti*. This recipe is for raw zucchini spaghetti noodles (zoodles), a low-carb, gluten-free, and vegetarian recipe. **Zucchini** itself is a fruit, but in culinary contexts it is treated as a vegetable. It is rich in water (about 90%) and is therefore very good for you during the hotter seasons and as part of a **weight loss plan.**

Once prepared, spaghetti should be served immediately because, as zucchini is very rich in water, they quickly lose their freshness.

DESSERTS

APPLE AND RICOTTA CAKE

Total preparation time: **1 hour**
Baking time: **45–50 minutes**
Yield: **4–5 servings**

3 medium golden delicious apples
½ organic lemon, zest + juice
2/3 cup (140 g) granulated sugar + 2–3 tablespoons
2 medium eggs
1 teaspoon vanilla extract
2.5 oz (70 g) unsalted butter, melted
2/3 cup (170 g) creamy cow's milk ricotta
3 tablespoons milk
1¾ cups (250 g) pastry flour
2 scarce teaspoons (8 g) baking powder
Powdered sugar for decoration

1   Preheat the oven to 350°F (180°C). Butter and flour a 9 inch (23 cm) spring form pan and set oven rack to middle position.

2   Peel apples and cut into quarters. Remove core and finely slice. Add juice of half a lemon to prevent browning and 2–3 tablespoons of sugar.

3   In a bowl, cream eggs and sugar with an electric whisk until pale yellow in color. Add vanilla, lemon zest, and ricotta softened with 1 tablespoon of milk. Mix and add butter. Mix well.

4   Sift flour and baking powder together. Slowly add to batter, then add 1–2 tablespoons of milk. The batter should be creamy.

5   Mix two-thirds of apples into batter.

6   Scrape batter into the pan and gently level the top with a spatula. Add rest of the apples.

7   Bake for 45–50 minutes. Remove from oven and let cool on a cooling rack for 5–8 minutes. Remove from pan and let it cool completely on cooling rack. Before serving, spread a thin layer of powdered sugar on top.

MAMMA MIA!

Apples are old fruits, dating back to the Stone Age. Native to Asia Minor, apples occupy a uniquely prevalent place in history. Recall the apple of Adam and Eve, Isaac Newton's apple, and the golden apple of Paris. Today, apples are still used in many cultures because they are delicious and very **healthy**; Italians have a phrase, *"Una mela al giorno toglie il medico di torno,"* which means "an apple a day keeps the doctor away." This is due to the antioxidant **polyphenols** and the protective substances and fiber that an apple contains, which are especially present in the peel. My advice is to buy **organic apples** and eat them with the skin so that you can receive more of the apple's vital nutrients, which include vitamins (A, B and C), minerals (sodium, potassium, iron, calcium, zinc and phosphorus) and fiber, in particular pectin, a polysaccharide which helps regulate the digestive system, and lower blood pressure, glucose levels, and "bad" LDL-cholesterol. Apples are the perfect allies in maintaining **healthy weight**, because they are **low in calories**, **rich in fiber,** and **prevent water retention**.

BAKED PEARS WITH WINE AND STAR ANISE

Total preparation time: **45 minutes**
Baking time: **35–40 minutes**
Yield: **2 servings**

2 medium size organic Abate Fetel or Bosc pears
2–3 tablespoons of honey
½ (120 ml) red wine, like Reciotto Valpolicella, Brachetto
   Piemonte or any fruity red wine
1 cinnamon stick
2 whole clove buds
3–4 anise stars

1   Preheat the oven to 350°F (180°C) and set oven rack to middle
    position.

2   Wash pears under running cold water and pat dry with paper
    towels. Peel and cut each pear in half lengthwise with a sharp,
    clean knife, keeping stem but removing core.

3   Place in a ceramic baking pan. Add honey, wine, cinnamon
    sticks, clove buds, and anise stars. Bake in the oven for about
    35–40 minutes, turning two or three times. Check after 25
    minutes, as the length of time required for baking depends on
    the ripeness of your pears. When they are done, they should
    be tender but not mushy and lightly browned.

4   You can serve either warm or at room temperature with some
    sauce and strained whole yogurt. If you want to prepare a
    richer version, you can substitute yogurt with 1 scoop of
    vanilla ice cream.

MAMMA MIA!

Star anise is the star shaped fruit of an evergreen plant known scientifically as *Illicium verum*. Star anise has a licorice-like flavor and originates from Asia. Today, it is used in the Italian cuisine because it is rich in flavor and has medicinal properties that endow it with significant health benefits such as **anti-viral, anti-fungal, and anti-bacterial properties**. Star anise should be stored in an airtight container away from heat and light.

DRIED FRUIT STUFFED WITH CHEESE YOGURT

Preparation time: **5 minutes**
Yield: **2 servings**

6 pieces mixed dried fruit (figs, dates and apricots)
6 tablespoons cheese yogurt (see recipe on page 224)
1 teaspoon rum
6 walnut or pecan halves

1   Make a slit in the center of each fruit. Remove the pit from the dates and apricots, if necessary.

2   In a bowl, mix together cheese and rum.

3   Fill the center of each fruit generously with cheese and place a walnut halve over the filling.

MAMMA MIA!

This is a delicious dessert that combines the sweet flavor of dried fruit, the health value of nuts, and the creamy texture of cheese yogurt. You *can* satisfy your sweet tooth with nutrient-rich ingredients. When you buy dried fruit, make sure to read the labels, as some products have sugar added.

PASSITO WINE-SOAKED NECTARINES

Total preparation time: **12 minutes**
Cooking time: **7–8 minutes**
Yield: **2 servings**

3 organic ripe nectarines, thickly sliced
1⅓ cups (320 ml) *Passito* wine or other sweet wine
1–2 tablespoons brown sugar
2–3 tablespoons Greek yogurt, to serve

1   In a saucepan, add wine and sugar and bring to a simmer. Cook for a few minutes over medium heat to reduce.

2   Add nectarines and cook until nectarines are a little bit tender but not mushy, about 7–8 minutes.

3   Let cool and serve with Greek yogurt. If you use peaches, it is better to peel them.

MAMMA MIA!

Passito wine is made from white grapes that have been dried to concentrate their juice. The classic method dries clusters of grapes on mats of straw in the sun or on modern racks, though some hang up the grapes or leave them to dry on the vine. The result is a sweet wine suitable for dessert. The *Moscato Passito di Pantelleria* is one of the most well-known *Passiti*. Other famous *Passiti* include *Vin Santo* in Tuscany, *Recioto* around Verona (Veneto), and *Sciacchetrà* from Cinque Terre (Liguria).

CARAMELIZED PINEAPPLE

Total preparation time: **20 minutes**
Cooking time: **11 minutes**
Yield: **4 servings**

1 medium pineapple, cored and cut into 8 rings
2–3 tablespoons brown sugar
½ teaspoon cinnamon
1 cup (240 ml) cognac or rum
2 oz (60 g) unsalted butter
Greek yogurt, to serve

1   In a small bowl, mix cognac, brown sugar, and cinnamon.

2   In a large sauce pan, melt butter, and then add cognac mix.
    Bring to simmer over medium-high heat, stirring constantly.
    Reduce to medium-low heat and cook for 3–4 minutes.

3   Lay pineapple rings in the sauce and continue to cook over
    medium heat for about 8 minutes, flipping midway through.

4   Transfer to a serving plate. Drizzle sauce on the slices and top
    with yogurt.

MAMMA MIA!

Pineapple has a vibrant tropical flavor that balances out the acid taste of yogurt. It is **rich in vitamins (such as vitamin C), minerals (such as potassium), fiber, and bromelain that are is very helpful to digestion**. Several studies have shown that consumption of pineapple decreases the rate of obesity and inflammation, as well as promoting general health. I love it in my fruit salad for breakfast and by itself as a healthy snack.

CHOCOLATE-COVERED STRAWBERRIES

Preparation time: **15 minutes**
Cooling time: **40 minutes**
Yield: **2 servings**

16 large strawberries (about 6–7 oz or 170–200 g)
4.5 oz (125 g) dark chocolate (70%)
Equipment
Double boiler and sauce pan
Heatproof spatula
Toothpicks
Paper towels
A piece of Styrofoam

1   Rinse strawberries under cool running water and gently pat dry with paper towels. Strawberries need to be completely dry before dipping into the chocolate; otherwise, chocolate coating will not stick very well. Insert a toothpick into the top of each strawberry.

2   On a cutting board, cut chocolate in pieces. In a double boiler and saucepan, bring water to a simmer, then add chocolate and let melt, stirring occasionally with the spatula. Remove saucepan from heat. Let cool until the chocolate reaches a temperature of 115°F (45°C).

3   Dip one strawberry at a time in the chocolate, holding it by the toothpick. Twist and turn the strawberry in the chocolate to completely coat it. Be careful to leave a band of red strawberry at the top not covered by chocolate.

4   Let cool by turning upside down and inserting the toothpick into a piece of Styrofoam covered with paper towels. Let cool

for about 30–40 minutes, depending on the temperature of the room. You can place the strawberries in the fridge to speed up this process.

MAMMA MIA!

Strawberries are **superfoods**, packed with **anti-oxidants (such as vitamin C), minerals (such as potassium), and fiber (helpful in managing weight loss)**. Strawberries are a good food option for **weight loss,** as long as you are not adding them to ice creams or cakes. Instead, use them with healthy food options such as smoothies, yogurt, and oatmeal Strawberries also contain xylitol, a sweet substance that prevents the formation of dental plaque and kills the germs responsible for bad breath.

ITALIAN COOKIES:
"UGLY BUT GOOD"

Total Preparation time: **1 hour and 10 minutes**
Baking time: **55–60 minutes**
Yield: **About 13–15 cookies**

3 medium eggs, egg whites at room temperature
1 vanilla pod, seeds
½ scarce cup (90 g) granulated sugar
1½ cups (about 170 g) toasted hazelnuts

1   Preheat a ventilated oven to 260°F (130°C) and set oven rack to middle position.

2   Chop hazelnuts in a food processor at medium speed until you reach the consistency of a coarse granola. Set aside.

3   Place egg whites in a large bowl. Add vanilla seeds and start mixing with an electric mixer at medium speed for at least 10–12 minutes, until fluffy. Egg whites should already look very bubbly and translucent before introducing sugar to the mix.

4   Add ⅓ of the sugar and mix until it is well incorporated. Repeat twice until you finish all sugar. Don't worry about over-beating; once sugar is added, meringue can be whipped almost indefinitely.

5   With a spatula, gently fold the hazelnuts into egg whites.

6   Line a baking sheet with parchment paper. Place a heaping tablespoon of hazelnut dough onto the baking sheet, about 1 inch (2.5 cm) apart.

7   Bake cookies for 55–60 minutes (or even longer), until lightly brown on top and crispy inside.

8   Let cool on a cooling rack before serving. Cookies can be stored in an airtight container for up to 3–4 days.

MAMMA MIA!

Looks can be deceiving, goes the popular saying, and these *brutti ma buoni* (ugly but good) cookies are a clear example. These cookies are a **healthy choice**: **gluten-free, free of added fats, and rich in a lot of nutrients**. **Hazelnuts are superfoods** to add to your diet (see page 44). Additionally, **egg whites** are a good source of **high-quality protein without fat**. Of course, these *are* cookies, so some sugar is needed to complete the recipe, but only enough to let the flavor of the hazelnuts come through!

KIWI AND ORANGE CAKE

Total preparation time: **1 hour**
Baking time: **45–50 minutes**
Yield: **4–5 servings**

5 medium kiwi, peeled and finely sliced
1 medium organic orange, juice + zest
2/3 cup (140 g) granulated sugar
2 medium eggs
1 teaspoon vanilla extract
2.5 oz (70 g) unsalted butter, melted
½ cup (120 ml) plain yogurt
1 scarce tablespoon (10 g) baking powder
¼ teaspoon (1.5 g) baking soda
1 heaping cup (150 g) spelt flour or pastry flour
2/3 cup (95 g) corn starch or potato starch
Powdered sugar, for decoration

1   Preheat the oven to 350°F (180°C). Butter and flour a 9 in
    (about 23 cm) spring-form pan and set oven rack to middle
    position.

2   In a bowl, mix kiwi slices with orange juice and set aside.

3   In another bowl, cream sugar and eggs with an electric whisk
    until pale yellow. Add butter, vanilla extract, orange zest and
    yogurt. Mix well to blend all ingredients.

4   Sift flours, baking powder, and baking soda together and
    slowly add it to the batter. Add orange juice from kiwi, one
    spoonful at a time. Mix well; batter should be creamy

5   Scrape ⅓ of the batter into the pan and place the kiwi on top,
    equally distributed. Add the remaining batter.

6   Bake for 45–50 minutes until golden browned on top.

7   Remove from oven and let cool on a cooling rack for 5 minutes. Remove from pan and let it cool completely on a cooling rack. Before serving, dust with a thin layer of powdered sugar.

MAMMA MIA!

This delicious dessert is one of my winter favorites—sweet, but with a tart flavor typical of kiwi and citrus. **Kiwi** are excellent sources of **vitamin C**, a water-soluble antioxidant which neutralizes free radicals. Free radicals can cause damage to cells and lead to problems such as inflammation and cancer. Kiwi are also **rich in minerals** such as potassium (a good ally against water retention) and fiber.

Kiwi's **vitamin C content** improves digestibility, fatigue recovery, intestinal function, and skin care, making it quite attractive—it makes you **healthier and beautiful** at the same time.

LEMON AND ROSEMARY SORBET

Total preparation time: **50 minutes + 8 hours freezing**
Cooling time: **8 hours**
Yield: **4–5 servings**

1 cup (240 ml) water
¾ cup (150 g) sugar
3 large organic lemons, filtered lemon juice
1 sprig rosemary, plus some for decoration
1 organic lemon, zest
1 teaspoon (5 g) carob seed flour
1 pasteurized egg white, at room temperature

1　Cool a steel bowl in the freezer for 30 minutes.

2　In a saucepan, combine sugar (reserving 4 teaspoons) and water and bring to boil over medium heat. Cook for 5 minutes, stirring continuously, until sugar is dissolved and mixture starts to simmer. Add lemon zest and rosemary. Remove from heat and cool completely. Filter out the zest and rosemary from sugar syrup. Let cool.

3　Mix 2 teaspoons of sugar and carob seed flour in a small bowl. Add ¼ cup sugar syrup and mix well with a whisk. In a separate bowl, beat egg white with an electric whisk. As soon it gets fluffy, add 2 teaspoons sugar and beat for 2 minutes.

4　Pour sugar syrup into the chilled bowl and stir in lemon juice and carob seed mixture. Add egg white and mix well. You can expect egg white to separate somewhat from lemon juice; that's normal.

5　For the final step, choose from two different methods:
Ice cream method: Pour mixture into an ice cream maker and follow the manufacturer's instructions.

Freezer method: My preferred method, Pour the mixture in a suitable container and store in the freezer for 1 hour. Remove and mix with a fork. Put back in the freezer for at least 3 hours. Remove from freezer, stir, and put back in the freezer for another 3–4 hours.

6   Place a few rosemary needles (finely chopped) in a cold blender jar and blend for just a few seconds. Add sorbet and blend for a few seconds to give it a creamy texture.

7   Freeze again for about 20 minutes. Decorate with rosemary needles (optional). You can also let it thaw a little bit and serve in a flute with a straw. Store in the freezer in an airtight container for several weeks.

MAMMA MIA!

This is a perfect summer treat, refreshing and beautifully light. You can serve it either as a dessert, a snack, or as a palate cleanser between courses. **Sorbet** is an ancient dessert; the Greeks thought it was the nectar of the gods, the Romans loved it too, and we are still enjoying it today in the 21st century! Sorbet is a frozen dessert *prepared* with sugar syrup and flavored with a variety of different fragrant fruit juices, fresh herbs (such as rosemary, basil, or mint), wine (champagne), and liqueur. Sorbet should have a soft and smooth texture, so I've added natural stabilizers to the recipe (such as carob seed flour and beaten egg white) instead of chemicals and milk products like the mass production industry uses. **Carob seed flour** is a **natural thickening agent**, rich in fiber, minerals, and protein. Egg white is rich in protein, too. Both improve the texture by decreasing the mixture's freezing point.

SEASONAL
MENUS

I T'S SO EASY NOWADAYS to forget about the role that seasons play in the foods we eat! With modern processing and worldwide distribution of food, a large variety of foods are available year-round; we can find the same foods in December that we do in August. Seeds can be sown indoors throughout the year in temperature and light controlled environments; herbicides and pesticides keep enemies away from crops in summer, allowing winter and spring foods to continue growing throughout the year; and, of course, summer foods such as stone fruit and tropical fruit are imported from abroad, incurring import taxes and freight charges. Consuming these foods that have been grown out of season can add unnecessary costs to our grocery bill; the special efforts that have been made in order to ensure availability usually include costs passed on to the consumer.

Still, it's important to celebrate the foods that are in their proper season, because that's when you'll find them at their most flavorful and nutritious. It is those fruits and vegetables that have been grown in their original season, have been properly ripened, and were most recently harvested which provide the best flavor and are at their nutritional peak. Therefore, to enjoy the full nourishment of food and to benefit from a food's nutritional potential, we must make our menu a seasonal one. Also, changing our palate with the seasons gives us a wider variety of food to enjoy, keeping us constantly interested in our meals while ensuring we don't accidentally cause nutritional deficiencies. Try to learn what foods grow in your region during the different seasons!

I have provided four sample menus which follow the Italian seasons to give an example of what I usually eat during the year, all while eating a MMD-friendly diet. However, in different parts of the world (and even in different regions of one country), seasonal menus can vary. In the recipes section you will find different recipes to prepare in different periods of the year. Feel free to adjust these menus according to the availability of fresh and seasonal ingredients in your own country.

A DAY IN WINTER

When you get up	A glass of warm water with the juice of half a lemon
Breakfast	Black coffee, cappuccino, or tea A slice of oatmeal and banana cake* A piece of fresh fruit
Morning snack	Freshly squeezed orange juice. Use two oranges and add two tablespoons of the remaining pulp back in
Lunch	Baby Spinach and Pomegranate Salad* Minestrone with Barley*
Afternoon snack	Plain yogurt (1 serving ½ cup, or 120 ml) with diced kiwifruit mixed in
Dinner	Mixed green salad with carrots and a tablespoon of mixed seeds Marinated Chicken Breast with Orange and Pistachios* Steamed basmati rice (1 serving = 1/4 cup or 45 g) Sautéed Brussels sprouts

The recipes marked with a star can be found in Part III: Recipes

A DAY IN SPRING

When you get up	A glass of warm water with the juice of half a lemon
Breakfast	Black coffee, cappuccino, or tea 1–2 slices of Whole Grain Italian Bread* with Homemade Low Sugar Jam* A glass of milk (cow's milk, almond milk, or soy milk) (1 serving = ½–3/4 cup or 120–180 ml)
Morning snack	A small handful of unsalted nuts (7–8, depending on type)
Lunch	Italian Salad * Buckwheat Pasta with Spinach and Prawns*
Afternoon snack	2 slices of fresh pineapple (cut whole or half pineapple for the family to share)
Dinner	Arugula salad with cherry tomatoes Baked Vegetable Frittata* 1 slice of Whole Grain Italian Bread*

* The recipes marked with a star can be found in Part III: Recipes

A DAY IN SUMMER

When you get up	A glass of water with the juice of half a lemon and some mint leaves
Breakfast	Black coffee or tea 1 Peach Shake* (1 serving = 3/4 cup or 180 ml) ½ slice of toasted Whole Grain Italian Bread*
Morning snack	1 slice of watermelon
Lunch	Grilled eggplant Chickpea Salad * 1 slice of Whole Grain Italian Bread*
Afternoon snack	Lemon and Rosemary Sorbet* (1 serving = ½ cup or 120 ml)
Dinner	Cucumber, tomatoes and olives salad ("Greek" salad) Codfish with Ginger and Pine Nuts* Steamed basmati rice (1 serving = ¼ cup or 45 g)

* The recipes marked with a star can be found in Part III: Recipes

A DAY IN AUTUMN

When you get up	A glass of warm water with the juice of half a lemon
Breakfast	Black coffee, cappuccino, or tea Plain, whole grain muesli, no sugar or fruit added (1 serving = ½ cup or 60 g) with yogurt and diced fruit
Morning snack	Freshly squeezed orange juice in 1 serving seasonal fruit (like pear)
Lunch	Fennel and Orange Salad* Pasta with Kale and Ricotta*
Afternoon snack	2 small squares of dark chocolate, 70% cocoa (approximately 1 oz or about 30 g)
Dinner	Mixed green salad with cherry tomatoes Beef Fillet with Mushrooms* Sautéed broccoli

* The recipes marked with a star can be found in Part III: Recipes

APPENDIX A

Cooking Techniques

"Eating is a necessity, but cooking is an art." And, like all arts, cooking requires certain knowledge regarding materials and techniques.

The art of preparing food and the cooking techniques involved vary across the world, depending on cultural traditions and economic development. Cooking is based primarily on chemistry: you start with ingredients and, through different cooking techniques, you create a final product that is completely different from the initial one. The only difference is that the products of experiments in the kitchen are almost always tastier than the ones in the lab!

There are plenty of ways to prepare and cook delicious dishes. In this section, we'll be giving an overview of the various cooking methods used in the Mamma Mia Diet, as well as an explanation of their effects on taste and nutritional content.

NO COOKING: WHEN AND WHY RAW IS GOOD

Fruits and Vegetables

Is it always better to eat fruits and vegetables raw?

The answer is … yes *and* no! Almost all fruits and vegetables maintain their full nutrient profile (vitamins, minerals and antioxidants) and support optimal health when eaten raw. However, some studies have found that cooking can amplify the bioavailability of certain nutrients present in vegetables, like lycopene in tomatoes and antioxidants and carotenoids in carrots, pumpkin, and peppers. Heat facilitates the release of nutrients by breaking down cell walls, providing an easier passage of nutrients from the food to the body.

Raw Fish, Meat and Eggs

It is better to eat fish, meat, and eggs cooked because these foods may carry parasites. In the case of fish, prior to consuming raw it must be frozen at specific temperatures and stored frozen for a certain period of time in order to effectively kill parasites. The internal temperature should be -4°F (or -20°C) for at least four days to kill any parasite that may be present. If you find a recipe that calls for raw eggs, avoid this recipe or use pasteurized eggs instead.

MARINATING: THE "EXTRA" FLAVOR

Marinating is a versatile technique. It boosts the flavor of meat and fish and even some vegetables and fruit. Marinating refers to soaking food in a flavorful liquid called a **marinade**, typically made of vinegar, lemon juice, wine, or yogurt with some spices and herbs. Always marinate meat and fish in the refrigerator.

When marinating fish, the acid in a marinade may appear to "cook" raw fish, leading some to wonder whether marinated fish can be eaten raw. However, despite appearances, marinating doesn't eliminate bacteria the same way cooking with heat does. When marinating fish that won't be cooked, make sure the fish is sushi-grade, or frozen-at-sea fish; both are safe for healthy adults to consume raw (however, it is not recommended for children, elderly people, or pregnant women).

BOILING

Boiling is a quick and easy method that has been used in many cultures for centuries. All you need is water and salt, depending on what you are cooking. The large volume of water and the high temperature dissolves many water-soluble nutrients, like water soluble vitamins (such as vitamin C and B) and minerals (such as potassium), but also makes some nutrients more digestible (such as starch).

Boiling Vegetables

While many vegetables are primarily eaten raw (such as lettuce, arugula, and cucumber), some need to be cooked, as they are unhealthy if consumed raw (such as potatoes, eggplant, legumes, pumpkin, and asparagus). Others can be prepared both ways (such as tomatoes, carrots, peppers, and spinach), depending on the recipe. When you boil vegetables, it is better to add them to hot salted water (except for potatoes; in this case, cold salted water is better to start with). When you cook legumes, start with unsalted cold water; otherwise they will be tough, because salt prevents hydration. Add salt only five minutes before removing them from the heat, to add some flavor.

Blanching and Steaming

Blanching is a cooking method wherein the food—typically a vegetable or fruit—is heated in boiling water, removed after a brief interval, and then plunged into iced water. Steaming is a cooking method that uses steam. Both of these are better methods for many vegetables because they preserve many nutrients.

Boiling Meat and Fish

In the case of boiling meat, you have to make a choice between having tasty meat and a rich stock. When I want tasty boiled meat, I put the meat in boiling water with some vegetables, such as carrots, onions, garlic and celery. However, if I want a tasty and rich stock, I place the meat in cold water. Using this method, most of the protein, vitamins and minerals gets dissolved in the stock.

When cooking fish in hot water, boiling for no longer than 20 minutes will not reduce the amount of omega-3 fatty acids, but you will lose some protein and vitamins in the water. However, fish is not a good source of vitamins, so they should not be your only source of vitamins during your meal. Additionally, most people already consume enough protein, so minimal protein loss should not be a deterrent for you to cook fish in water.

PRESSURE COOKING

Food cooked in a pressure cooker requires very little water and time, which means that vitamins and minerals are kept intact. The cooker seals in steam, created by the boiling liquid, which increases flavor. A whole chicken can be ready in fifteen minutes; rice in five minutes, and most vegetables in about three minutes. This method was used a lot in Italy before microwaving became popular. I grew up with a pressure cooker in our family kitchen, and I still use it today, mainly to cook vegetables. For soups, stews, and other ingredients I prefer other healthy traditional methods. After all, a good cook likes to check all the steps of cooking, and I am naturally curious!

GRILLING

Grilling is a great cooking method, requiring minimal additions of fat and imparting a smoky flavor while keeping meat, fish, and veggies juicy and tender. This is an excellent method of cooking in a weight losing plan, but like everything, it is not perfect and can be harmful to your health when used inappropriately.

Grilling Fruits and Vegetables

Grilled vegetables are an appetizing and tasty side dish, ideal to prepare for a cookout. Grilling is a healthy method of cooking that preserves flavor, most nutrients (when grilled for a short time without burning) and enhances the taste of fresh vegetables like tomatoes, zucchini, eggplant, onions, and bell peppers, as well as fruits such as mango, pineapple, and apple.

Grilling Meat and Fish

Grilled meat is certain a tasty food, but the smoky flavor and the char that you get from well-grilled meat is not particularly good for you. When fat from the cooking meat drips down on the hot coals, the smoke formed contains polycyclic aromatic hydrocarbons (PAHs). Cooking at high heat can also produce a chemical reaction between the fat and protein in meat, creating toxins that are linked to imbalance the antioxidants in the body. In addition, the charred exterior of the meat, when it is particularly dark, is full of heterocyclic amines (HCAs). Some research suggests that **regularly consuming charred, well-done red meat may increase risk of colorectal, pancreatic, and prostate cancer.**[1]

Marinating lowers this risk by preventing the formation of some toxins. One simple ingredient that can make all the difference is

---

1 Alomirah et al., 2011

rosemary, a typical Mediterranean herb that it commonly used in Italian cuisine for grilling and roasting. Studies show that adding it to ground beef and other types of muscly meat before grilling, frying, or broiling significantly reduces HCAs.

What does all this mean for you? While BBQs needn't necessarily be forbidden, I would recommend you choose lean cuts of meat that require less cooking time, keep dark meats on the rarer side, use marinades with herbs, flip meat every minute or so, and, when you can, use a cast-iron grill pan over a charcoal grill. Another idea is to cook your meat in an oven and then finish over the grill. This minimizes the grill exposure time, but you will still have the delicious flavor that is characteristic of grilled foods.

Fish is delicious on a grill, too, but you have to use the same precautions as with meat (no burning, marinades with herbs and preferring a cast-iron grill). Most fish is rich in omega-3 fatty acids that are minimally affected by grilling. In fact, studies have found no evidence of difference in omega-3 fatty acids composition when salmon was raw, poached, steamed, grilled, or baked.

FRYING

Stir-Frying

Stir-frying is a cooking technique in which ingredients are fried in a small amount of hot oil while being stirred in a nonstick cast-iron pan or wok. This quick, hot cooking method seals in the flavors of foods, as well as preserving their color and texture. It is good for vegetables cut in small pieces, as well as poultry and fish.

Deep Frying

Fried food should not be consumed on a regular basis, but once in a while, you are allowed to enjoy it. However, it is best to fry at home using some of the following tips:

 Choose the right fat at the right temperature.

 Cut food into small pieces. Cooking time will be faster and most of the nutritional value will be preserved. However, smaller pieces of food have an increased surface area, meaning that the food will absorb more of the oil and more of the oxidized products, which will add more calories and potentially harmful products to your food. Therefore, be fast!

3 Place a few pieces at a time into the hot oil, instead of the whole bunch all at once. Food will cook faster and will be crunchier.

4 Change fat as soon as it gets brown and starts to smoke. At this point, toxic compounds are being produced.

5 As soon as fried food is done, place on paper towels, but don't cover; this will remove excess fat.

6 Don't burn fried food. Acrylamide is a toxic chemical compound that forms during the cooking process in many of the starchy foods we love, like potatoes, breads, cookies, cakes, and coffee—especially when they are fried, baked, roasted, and broiled. Acrylamide is genotoxic and carcinogenic in animal studies, though results from human studies have provided only limited and inconsistent evidence of increased risk of developing cancer.[2] Acrylamide is created when a sugar and an amino acid called asparagine combine during high-temperature cooking or heating for extended lengths of time. This means that avoiding frying or otherwise burning or charring foods is an effective way to cut down the exposure.

---

2 EFSA, 2015

For more information about deep frying and better fat to use, refer
to Chapter 5: Fat and the Mamma Mia Diet.

BAKING

Baking is an antique method of cooking that uses prolonged dry
heat, normally from an oven, but also in hot ashes or on hot stones.
The most common baked items are bread, cakes, cookies, and, of
course, pizza, as well as meat, fish, fruits, and vegetables. I bet everyone remembers the smell of freshly baked bread; it makes us kids
again!

Baking Vegetables

Unfortunately, baking vegetables can destroy heat-sensitive vitamins, including vitamin C and some B vitamins. If you use fluids
such as stock during the cooking process, water-soluble vitamins
may be lost (unless the liquid is consumed with the food). A good
trick is baking in parchment paper, or *cottura al cartoccio* in Italian.
This method involves wrapping food (mainly vegetables and fish)
in parchment paper and then baking it in the oven for a short time
at 375°F (180°C). This method is very easy, healthy, and impressive.
This method does not require much fat because the food effectively
steams inside the parchment paper.

Baking Meat and Fish

While baked meat and fish definitely taste good and are healthy, be
careful not to brown them. Baking usually requires little added fat,
and if you use a roasting rack, any fat will drain out during cooking.

Baking fish preserves most of nutrients, including the omega-3
fatty acids . Baking fish *en papilotte*, in parchment paper, also keeps
is moist and flavorful.

MICROWAVING

Microwaving is a cooking technique that I personally prefer to avoid because I cannot see the food transformations during the cooking process; for me, it is like cooking in the dark. However, it is a very rapid method for when you don't have time to do anything else. Food cooks very fast through an increase of temperature due to the effect of electromagnetic waves.

There are many controversial studies about the overall safety of microwave ovens; some people believe further studies will reveal evidence of microwaves harming humans; others enjoy the time-saving convenience a microwave oven offers. Therefore, using a microwave is a personal choice.

When cooking vegetables, this method offers no advantages from a nutritional point of view over steaming; it's just faster. When cooking meat and fish, microwave cooking is similar to pan cooking, only faster. Finally, as regards pasta and rice, the amount of time needed to cook in a microwave isn't significantly faster than traditional preparation methods ... and let's face it, for an Italian to cook pasta in the microwave is a sin!

APPENDIX B

The Secret of Pasta

Pasta, the **queen** ingredient of **Italian cuisine**, is known and loved all over the world and is a staple of the Italian diet. But do you know why?

Pasta is **healthy**, tasty and easy to prepare. Usually prepared as a mixture of durum wheat flour and water, which is then dried and cut into various shapes, pasta can also be produced with other grains, and eggs may be used instead of water. Pasta is a source of **good carbohydrates** (about 79.1 g per 3.5 oz or 100 g dried pasta) which serve as one of the body's primary sources of fuel. Pasta is also a discrete source of **B vitamins and protein** (10–12 g per 3.5 oz or 100 g dried pasta) and is good source of **minerals**, while being **low in sodium** and **cholesterol free**. Whole grain pasta also provides a beneficial amount of fiber that can reduce the risk of developing metabolic diseases related to unhealthy diet.

Provided it's consumed in reasonable portions, pasta is absolutely the type of ingredient that should be present in one's diet. In traditional large Italian meals, pasta dishes are served as a first course (*primo*) and the portions are small because the servings are sometimes followed by a second course (*secondo*), usually meat or fish, which by itself might often be considered a full meal. The MMD suggests serving pasta as the main course, preceded by a salad.

DIFFERENT PASTA CATEGORIES

Pasta can be divided in **two major categories**: **dried pasta (pasta secca)**, which is made with durum wheat flour or other grains flours; and **fresh pasta (pasta fresca)**, which is prepared with soft wheat flour (or Italian grade oo flour, very similar to pastry flour or unbleached all-purpose flour) and eggs. The eggs enhance the yellow color of the pasta, reduce stickiness, and improve its elasticity, which is especially valuable for longer pasta shapes such as *tagliatelle*.

Most dried pasta is made industrially in large quantities, but a few artisanal producers still make it the traditional way, often using **old grains** such as Senatore Cappelli, Kamut, Grano monocco, and many others that are **not GMOs** (genetically modified organisms). Their method uses bronze extrusion dies (which are perforated plates used for shaping), and the pasta is dried slowly at low temperatures. Consequently, artisanal pasta has a rough and porous texture (which allows sauces to cling better) and it usually *"mantiene bene la cottura"* (meaning it keeps its *al dente* texture longer). This method makes Italian pasta something unique, different in its quality and taste from the pasta produced in other ways and in other countries.

Available in a variety of formats and paired with countless tasty sauces, our pasta is something that we Italians are very proud of.

Pasta Shapes

On the topic of pasta and sauce, it is very important to pair the 'right' pasta shape with the 'right' sauce. Smooth sauces are fine for long pasta (like spaghetti) where the sauce flows around the noodles, while chunky sauces call for concave-shaped pasta or one with holes (like *penne* or *maccheroni*). Certain short pasta (*farfalle* and *fusilli*) are also good to be served cold (like in pasta salad), as it keeps its texture for a long time.

Sauce should be served in proportional amounts to the pasta; it should not "smother" the pasta. The pasta must always remain the star of the show.

I group pasta shapes into **five general categories**:

1 Short pasta (Ex.: *penne, farfalle, fusilli, maccheroni, orecchiette*)

2 Long pasta (Ex.: *spaghetti, bucatini, linguine,* noodles, angel hair, *tagliatelle*)

3 Filled pasta (Ex.: *tortellini, ravioli, cannelloni*)

4 Lasagna

5 Pasta for soups (Ex.: such as thimbles, bells, rings)

The main purpose of having different pasta shapes is to hold the sauce better, whatever that sauce may be. The shape may also be determined depending on the roughness of the dough. You'll find that pasta shapes differ greatly from north to south; this is due to the different sauces prepared in these regions using the ingredients available in different climates. In the south, where the climate is warmer, olive oil, tomatoes, fresh vegetables, olives, capers, and seafood are staples. In the north, however, where the climate is colder and more humid, cheese, butter, and cream are frequently used to prepare sauces.

HOW TO COOK PASTA

Cooking time for pasta depends both on the format and the type of pasta. It is usually 11–12 minutes for pasta *secca* (dried pasta), because the pasta needs to rehydrate; cooking time is shorter for fresh pasta—for example, *tagliatelle* which will take about 3–4 minutes, or *ravioli*, which takes 4–5 minutes.

When cooking pasta, there are four key "ingredients":

Water. For every 3.5 oz (100 g) of pasta, you need about 1 quart (1 liter) of water. Pasta should be cooked in a large pan, since pasta tends to stick if cooked in a small pan. The normal portion size per person is about 2.5–3 oz (about 70-80 g), about which comes to about 250–280 calories.

Salt. The ratio of salt to water is very important. Chefs recommend around 2 rounded scarce teaspoons of sea salt for every quart (liter) of water. If the pasta sauce has a strong seasoning, the amount of salt should be reduced proportionately. It might be that very little salt is necessary; for example, if pasta is served with pesto, which can be quite salty by itself, you won't find it necessary to add much salt to the cooking water. **I always add very little salt to my pasta (less than a teaspoon per 1 quart of water). I recommend a low salt diet; it is much healthier!** Just remember that it is important to adjust the amount of salt to the type of sauce.

The ideal time to add salt to water is after it starts boiling to reduce the boiling time; if you add salt to cold water, the time to boil will be longer. This step, however, is not critical; adding it early just results in a few minutes' difference.

Most of the time, to prevent pasta from sticking, people will add 1–2 tablespoons of oil to the water during cooking. I don't like to do that because pasta will become oily itself and, as a result, the sauce will slide off without getting absorbed—no to mention the pasta itself will be flavorless. Instead, for the first couple minutes, you should stir the pasta. Stirring at the beginning will keep the pasta from sticking to itself.

Time. Pasta should not be soft or mushy when it is served. Cooking should be *al dente*—literally translated as "to the tooth," which means that the cooked dough should be firm and have a bit of resistance when you bite into it. **Pasta al dente** is tastier and healthier because it helps keep blood sugar stable.

To test whether your pasta is done, halve your noodle and view the inside; when the color is uniform but with just a white spot in the center, your pasta is just right—*al dente*—as opposed to when the entire inside is still white, meaning the pasta is not cooked enough. Remember that pasta will continue to cook for a short time after it is drained. I would recommend draining your pasta while it is still just slightly underdone, making it perfectly *al dente* when you eat it. After you drain pasta, you should *not* rinse under cold water (unless you are preparing a cold pasta salad), because you will remove the absorbent surface and the sauce will not cling to the pasta properly.

Sauce. Before draining the pasta, reserve some cooking water to add to the pasta and sauce. The amount of cooking water depends on the recipe (usually about ¼ cup or 60 ml). Drain pasta and pour it in the pan with the sauce. Add cooking water and mix gently. This is the final moment of preparation. Let it heat for one minute on high heat, and then serve immediately.

And that's the way we, in Italy, prepare pasta.

APPENDIX C
Conversion Tables

All recipes have imperial and metric measurements. The accuracy and correctness of the conversions are suitable for cooking, but not for scientific purposes. In any case, bear in mind, for example, that two ingredients measured in volume will have differing weights. For example, 1 cup flour, which weighs about 140 g, versus 1 cup of sugar, which weighs about 200 g, since they have different weights for the same volume.

Refer to the table below for approximate conversion rations; in the recipes the numbers may have been rounded for ease of reference.

METRIC	IMPERIAL		
Volume (Liquid Ingredients)		112 g	4 oz
0.950 ml	1 qt	56 g	2 oz
237 ml	1 c	28 g	1 oz
177 ml	¾ c	Length	
118 ml	½ c	2.5 cm	1 inch
80 ml	⅓ c		
60 ml	¼ c		
30 ml	⅛ c		
15 ml	1 tablespoon		
5 ml	1 teaspoon		
Weight (Dry Ingredients)			
900 g	32 oz		
450 g	16 oz/1 pound		
225 g	8 oz		

ABBREVIATIONS

oz = ounce
°F = degrees Fahrenheit
cm = centimeter
g = gram
ml = milliliter
l = liter
°C = degrees Centigrade

ACKNOWLEDGEMENTS

The work of an author is not a solitary experience. There are always those people who play a critical role in the creation of a masterpiece, who all too often remain unknown to the readers.

Therefore, I would like to express my special thanks to my husband and my children for their support and encouragement throughout the production of this book.

My special thanks are extended to my colleague Paola Palestini for her valued collaboration. Paola is a very enthusiastic and professional person who accompanied me in this journey. I thoroughly enjoyed working with her and am happy that she agreed to help me with this project.

Thank you to Andrew Flach, my publisher, for trusting me and encouraging me; Ryan Tumambing, for his technical assistance; and Anna Krusinski and Ryan Kennedy, for their wonderful job in editing this book.

My thanks are extended to Elena Bianchi, my personal photographer, for her impressive and appetizing food photography. I would also like to thank Katharine McKeever and Christine Richardson for their kind and valuable contributions in editing some parts of the book.

Thank you to the readers of my blog and my followers; without them, I would not be here writing my second book.

Last, but not least, I am grateful to my friend Sue McGregor for her constructive suggestions. Her willingness to give her time so generously has been very much appreciated.
   —**Paola Lovisetti Scamihorn**

I would like to thank the two men in my life—my husband Bruno and my son Edoardo—for having supported me in these months of writing; my mother, Rosanna, and my aunt, Iaia, who taught me to cook; my Lab's Biochemistry Girls for their significant scientific contribution; and last but not least, my present and future students, for the constant motivation to be the best!
   —**Paola Palestini**

ABOUT THE AUTHORS

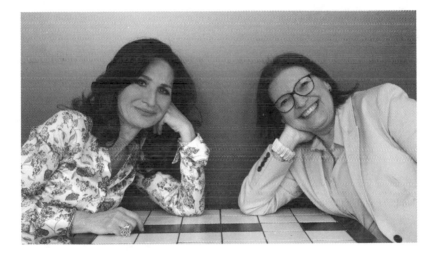

Paola Lovisetti Scamihorn is an Italian pharmacist, researcher and food writer. Cooking, eating healthy food and staying active have always been her life-long passions. She has a cooking blog "Passion and Cooking," and contributes to several international magazines. She has previously published in Italy Love is Eating, focusing on Italian culinary culture.

Paola Palestini is a biochemistry professor at the Medical School of the University Milano-Bicocca, Italy. Recently, Paola has been actively involved in the promotion of the principles of a healthy diet through conferences and in collaboration with several magazines. She is the author of seventy-six scientific articles published in international journals.

SELECTED BIBILIOGRAPHY

CHAPTER 2

1. Daniel and Tollefsbol, 2015

2. Hardy and Tollefsbol, 2011

3. Sanz, 2016

CHAPTER 3

4. Lustig, 2010

5. Kolderup and Svihus, 2015

6. Huang et al., 2016

7. USDA, Dietary Guidelines for Americans: 6th, 2015, USDA. Dietary Guidelines for Americans: 7th, 2015.

8. Albertson et al., 2016

9. Serra-Majem and Bautista-Castano, 2015

10. Reilly, 2016

11. A complete GI table for more than 1,000 foods can be found in the article "International tables of Glycemic Index and glycemic load values" Atkinson et al., 2008.

12. Chiu et al., 2011

13. Temelkova-Kurktschiev et al., 2000

CHAPTER 4

14. U.S. Department of Health and Human Services and U.S. Department of Agriculture. 2015–2020

15. Mayne et al., 2016

16. Kim and Kim 2015; Martí et al., 2016

17. Kushi et al., 1999; Curran, 2012

18. Afshin et al., 2014

19. Vuksan et al., 2017

CHAPTER 5

20. Mozaffarian, 2016

21. Säemann MD et al., 2000

22. Pes GM et al., 2015

23. Zong G.et al, 2016

24. Richardson et al. 2017

25. Richardson et al., 2017

26. Clarke et al., 1997; Jensen et al., 1999

27. Mukherjee and Mitra 2009; Marangoni et al., 2017

28. Cardoso et al. 2015

29. KudaO, 2017

30. ShiZ et al., 2016

31. Blasbalg et al. 2011

CHAPTER 6

32. Hecker, 2001

33. Yan and Spitznagel, 2009; Messina, 2014.

34. Chao, 2008

35. Bernstein et al., 2015

36. Bernstein et al., 2015

37. Stamler, 1979; Yusuf et al., 2004

38. Newby et al., 2005

39. Campa et al., 2012

40. Craig ct al., 2009

41. Melnik et al., 2016

42. Bouglé and Bouhallab , 2017

43. Italian LARN, 2014

44. Tai et al., 2015

45. Crowe et al., 2008; Pala et al., 2011; Murphy et al., 2013

46. Handelman et al., 1999

47. Howell et al., 1997

CHAPTER 7
48. Fang et al., 2015

CHAPTER 8
49. Samihah Zura Mohd Nani et al., 2016

50. Renaud and de Lorgeril, 1992

51. Grønbaek et al., 2000

52. Arteroa et al., 2015

53. Arteroa et al., 2015

54. Bertelli, 2005

55. Gertsch, 2011

56. IARC Working Group on the Evaluation of Carcinogenic Risks to Humans, 2010

57. Ohnishi and Razzaque, 2010

58. Helm and Macdonald, 2015

59. Chen et al., 2010

60. Cano-Marquina et al., 2013

61. Souza et al., 2017

62. Sanchis-Gomar et al., 2016

63. Barrense-Dias, 2016

64. Rossheim et al., 2016; Lalanne et al., 2107

65. Robins et al., 2016

CHAPTER 10

66. St-Onge et al., 2017

67. Hutchinson et Heilbronn, 2016

CHAPTER 11

68. Jayne et al., 2014

CHAPTER 12

69. Wu et Zhai, 2014

CHAPTER 13

70. Rahman et al., 2013

71. Pallavi and Rathai, 2015

72. Medagama, 2015

73. Shah et al., 2011

74. Patil et al., 2016

75. Aggarwal 2010; Pulido-Moran et al., 2016

76. Türközü and Tek, 2017

77. Kraemer et al., 2002

78. Hunter et al., 2008

79. Hansen et al., 2005

APPENDIX A

80. Alomirah et al., 2011

81. EFSA, 2015